Praise for *Looking Past Dementia*

Looking Past Dementia offers a much-needed new vision of caring for people living with dementia. With its compelling stories and solid advice gleaned from Marysue Moses's long career working in memory care settings, this book could take the place of hours of dull lectures about dementia. As I read it, I imagined sending a copy to every person working in memory care, including administrators and marketing people, activities directors, nurses, CNAs, cooks, housekeepers, maintenance people, etc. I also thought about the many family caregivers I know who could use a gentle reminder that people living with dementia don't lose the ability to give and receive love. This beautiful work reverberates with messages of hope and offers multiple examples of how joy and meaning can be retained when we honor the humanity of people living with dementia by "looking past" their brain changes and acknowledging they have much to teach us.

—**Susan H. McFadden, PhD,** Professor Emerita of Psychology, cofounder of Fox Valley Memory Project, and coauthor of *Dementia-Friendly Communities*

Looking Past Dementia by Marysue Moses is a must-read for anyone working in dementia care. Marysue masterfully guides readers beyond the symptoms, losses and challenges associated with dementia to reveal the unique person who remains. Through her compassionate insights and real-world experience, she helps professionals and families understand not only how to provide better support, but also why so many of us are passionate about serving people living with dementia. This book reminds us that meaningful connections, genuine relationships, and opportunities for purpose continue long after a dementia diagnosis. Marysue beautifully captures what those of us in memory care know to be true: when we learn to look past dementia, we discover remarkable individuals whose lives still have tremendous value, wisdom and potential for connection. I highly recommend this book to healthcare professionals, caregivers and family members seeking a deeper understanding of person-centered dementia care.

—**Amy House,** host and owner of Think Dementia

As a geropsychologist working with dementia patients on a daily basis for forty-five years, I know firsthand that the quality of the relationships they have with caregivers and family members directly affected that their quality of life. Marysue Moses uses her years of experience working with these individuals to highlight the humanity, uniqueness and personality that remains in them despite their dementia diagnosis. She demonstrates how to touch people in an emotionally meaningful way. *Looking Past Dementia* should provide hope, encouragement and new ways of thinking for those who care for and love someone living with dementia.

—**John E. Brose, PhD,** CEO and clinical director of Associated Clinic of Psychology

Looking Past Dementia is a deeply moving book that reminds us that humor, love and humanity do not disappear with a dementia diagnosis. Marysue Moses offers hope, compassion and practical wisdom through personal stories and meaningful insights that caregivers, families and professionals can immediately connect with and apply. Her thoughtful guidance, including support for families navigating the transition into a memory care community, makes this book both an invaluable resource and an inspiring read. She has created a heartfelt reminder that dementia does not diminish the human spirit. My heart is happy reading this book! There's so much gloom surrounding a dementia diagnosis… *Looking Beyond Dementia* is proof that it does not have to be that way. With the right support, all those living with brain changes can thrive!

—**Melissa Elvrum,** founder of Creative Lucidity

Although the title of this book is *Looking Past Dementia*, Marysue Moses provides an invaluable roadmap for embracing its daily realities head-on with open arms and practical wisdom. The book is full of heartwarming, relatable and engaging true stories that vividly illustrate a wide range of experiences individuals living with dementia and their care partners encounter. Moses seamlessly shares practical strategies and tips she has learned through her years of dedicated work in the field. An easy and lighthearted read, the focus on positivity and promoting quality of life feels like a breath of fresh air.

—**Robyn Birkeland, PhD,**
dementia care research study interventionist

Whether you have family members with dementia or are starting to deal with it yourself, *Looking Past Dementia* will bring relief, insight and the ability to navigate the condition without panic. While experiencing her mother's illness, author Marysue Moses used her theater background to create respectful, effective approaches to communication and engagement that build understanding and connection. Moses's years of experience working in memory care serve her well here, and each chapter brings unexpected insights that make life easier for caregivers and loved ones. Ultimately, she teaches us not to be afraid of the losses we may endure, and that laughter, love and joy will remain part of our lives whether dementia happens or not. This book shares the journeys of many with this condition, while at the same time, offering ideas and support. You will be better prepared, happier and more informed for having read this wonderful book.

—**Jenna Zark,** author of *Crooked Lines* and the Beat Street Series, and family member of loved ones living with dementia

Looking Past Dementia is filled with wonderful insights from a professional with a true heart for those living with dementia and their caregivers. This book is a beautiful celebration of the unique talents of all those whose lives have been touched by dementia. It also teaches those involved in caregiving how to connect with and bring out these talents that are still inside—how to look past dementia—and enrich the lives of both the caregiver and the cared for. Kudos to Marysue Moses on *Looking Past Dementia*—a true gift to us all!

—**Marsha Brintnall,** daughter and sister of loved ones who lived with dementia

Marysue Moses is a wonderful dementia educator. Her book, *Looking Past Dementia*, provides insight into the experiences of those living with dementia. Her storytelling makes it easy to step into the lives of the people she writes about. As an executive director of a memory care community, I will be sharing this book with my team and the families we support.

—**Melissa Zentz,** executive director of memory care

LOOKING PAST DEMENTIA

LOOKING PAST DEMENTIA

Learning from Those Who Live with It

Marysue Moses

Foreword by Megan Carnarius

EMERALD LAKE BOOKS

Sherman, Connecticut

Looking Past Dementia:
Learning from Those Who Live with It

Shakespeare quotations are from the public-domain MIT Shakespeare edition of *The Complete Works of William Shakespeare* at shakespeare.mit.edu. Some quotations have been excerpted, and initial capitalization or terminal punctuation may have been adjusted for epigraph presentation.

Books published by Emerald Lake Books® may be ordered from your favorite booksellers or by visiting emeraldlakebooks.com.

Library of Congress Cataloging-in-Publication Data

Names: Moses, Marysue, 1952- author

Title: Looking past dementia : learning from those who live with it / Marysue Moses, MA.

Description: [Sherman] : Emerald Lake Books, [2026] | Includes bibliographical references.

Identifiers: LCCN 2026023184 (print) | LCCN 2026023185 (ebook) | ISBN 9781945847967 trade paperback | ISBN 9781945847974 epub

Subjects: LCSH: Dementia--Patients--Care | Dementia--Treatment | Dementia--Alternative treatment | Caregivers--Family relationships

Classification: LCC RC521 .M67 2026 (print) | LCC RC521 (ebook)

LC record available at https://lccn.loc.gov/2026023184

LC ebook record available at https://lccn.loc.gov/2026023185

First and foremost, to Margaret Coleman Moses.

And to all the other individuals living with dementia who have crossed my path and taught me well. Your names have been changed for privacy, but your spirits could never be disguised.

And to Phil and Eliza, the brightest lights I've known.

Table of Contents

Foreword

There are serendipitous moments that are meant to be, however mundane they seem at first. In 2014, while riding an airport shuttle bus headed to Denver from Boulder, Colorado, we stopped to pick up a passenger. She looked familiar. At that time, I was the director of a memory care residence nearby. She said, "Oh, hi Megan. I've been to many of your lectures. My mother has Alzheimer's and lives in a care community in Denver."

Marilyn introduced herself and told me that her sister, Marysue, had been a Memory Care Coordinator and was now the Dementia Program Coordinator for a company in Minnesota. When I am out and about in the world, it is very rare for me to run into someone else doing the same work, so I was intrigued. I asked if Marilyn would give her sister my contact information.

I had been working in this field for twenty-five years by the time Marysue and I connected in person. During that time, I provided direct management and operational support of memory care spaces, designed communities, seen them through construction, created all policies and procedures, and trained the staff. Marysue invited me to visit and deliver training and workshops for her teams. It was delightful and refreshing to meet someone who shared similar views and instincts about this work, and who was also busy helping care teams and families understand this wider and deeper wish for quality of life for the people we worked with. And so, I am excited to be a part of this moment of Marysue completing her book!

In *Looking Past Dementia*, Marysue Moses brings storytelling, insight and practical techniques to help us see the possibilities of creating a more fulfilling life for individuals with dementia. How can we connect? How can we build relationship? What brings joy and laughter? How can we keep love at the center of our intent? How can someone truly be seen, allowing that individual to be the focus more than the illness affecting them?

Marysue's breadth of understanding is evident in this book. She has captured so many important points about dementia care in this offering, illustrated with examples from her experience. Marysue is both highly observant and articulate. She is thoughtful and suggests different ways to respond to situations. As a reader, this experience-sharing pulls you in. Marysue is simultaneously humble and knowing, patient and urgent. She raises the bar on what's possible for individuals with memory loss.

Marysue shares insights and reactions directly from individuals in her care. We get to hear their voices and perceptions, and better understand the impact this dementia process has through the stories of residents who taught her or showed her important lessons. We have all had something special or unique happen with someone in our care. They might have said something profound, and we walk away saying, "Oh, I should write that down," then move on to the next thing. Marysue wrote them down!

This is a wonderful book for families navigating the dementia journey, who will benefit from the book's tone, stance and descriptions of this process. Marysue fully appreciates and conveys the poignancy of this journey, while supporting ways for families to remember and appreciate their loved one's strengths and emphasize what they can still do. *Looking Past Dementia* does not gloss over what is also difficult and changing, but allows more hope and space in the recognition of those things. Ultimately, we are invited to create meaning, honor emotions, and support well-being in the person with dementia in a way that makes sense to them.

This is also a wonderful book for caregiving professionals. It provides a treasure trove of tangible, applicable and immediate insights at our fingertips. In aging services, we talk about person-directed or person-centered care, and sometimes people don't really understand what that looks like. Marysue provides so many examples and suggestions, which I'm sure will inspire life enrichment staff and caregivers alike. She has also acknowledged and referenced numerous important contributors to this field, which can help expand our understanding. This book should be a primer for anyone going into this field of work and a refresher for any long-standing professional.

This valuable book comes at a time when dementia is viewed in such a negative and pessimistic light. It's the most dreaded disease for many people, especially older adults. Yet it is here among us, and we need to work with it, to find ways to overcome our biases and fears. For example, note the evolution in recent decades of society's view of disabilities. The use of the term "differently abled" instead of "disabled" shows an expansion of acceptance only dreamed of fifty years ago. Events like the Special Olympics and the athletes' amazing feats have helped in normalizing the absorption of differences while creating admiration for individuals who are overcoming obstacles and excelling beyond them.

In the current state of dementia caregiving, Marysue is a change agent, advocate and envelope pusher! She is a breath of fresh air, but also someone who has done the work and walks her talk. There is a genuine, authentic quality to what she is helping us see. She is illuminating the real opportunities to create more fulfilling lives for people living with dementia.

Marysue is a creative innovator and inspires us to be so as well. She models how to connect with the individuals around her and works hard to allow them to shine through. Listening for their insights helps create a better quality, more fulfilling life for these people. Marysue values their contributions and recognizes the potential in each person.

Reading this book, I laughed, cried, commiserated, applauded and appreciated how accessible Marysue made these experiences to us. Her synthesis is absorbable and applicable. We are lucky to be able to share and learn from her insights. I am grateful this will now be available to a wider, appreciative audience.

Megan Carnarius
Owner of Memory Care Consulting and author of
A Deeper Perspective on Alzheimer's and Other Dementias

Mom's Journey Begins

What change is this?
—William Shakespeare, *A Midsummer Night's Dream*, act 3, sc. 2

Margaret

Margaret awakens in the middle of the night, sits up straight, and stretches her right arm into the darkness. Her hand is still unfamiliar with the pathway to the switch on her new bedside lamp. After a bit of trial and error, she finds the base and sighs in relief. Her fingers fumble for the… *What's that called, anyway?* she wonders. *The thingy that you turn. Aha!* She finds the knob and twists it.

Once her eyes adjust to the brightness, Margaret surveys her surroundings. She feels out of place in the tiny apartment she moved into a few months ago. *What am I doing in this suffocating space? And where am I?* Neural activity deep within her brain is trying to remind her she is in Denver, Colorado, on the thirtieth floor of a senior high-rise, but she cannot decode that garbled message.

Never mind that. The question is: Where is my family? Though her son lives a few miles away and one of her four daughters is in Boulder, Margaret isn't thinking about them, and it's not her late husband she's missing now, either. She's longing for her father, mother and brothers. One thing feels certain: she needs to get home.

Margaret uses the bathroom, washes her hands and face, gets dressed, grabs her purse, and finds the elevator. It's a long ride down in that cold, metallic box. She is grateful when the doors slide open at last. All is eerie—too quiet—but the gentleman behind the front desk seems pleasant enough when he glances up from his book. Though he appears surprised to see her, he gives Margaret a warm smile as she approaches.

"Would you please call me a taxi?"

The man lifts his eyebrows and opens his mouth, yet no words come out.

Margaret hastens to explain. "I need to go home… to Junction City, Kansas."

Thankfully, the security guard was savvy enough to ensure Mom returned to her apartment and my Colorado siblings were notified.

Learning about dementia began with my mother, Margaret. No one in our family knew much about cognitive decline when Mom started to exhibit challenges in this arena. When my father died, she was close to seventy-five years old. In her bereavement, she rallied her forces, taking on the mountain of unfamiliar financial, legal and mundane tasks her conscientious husband had managed. Every morning, Mom made sure to get herself outdoors. She strode around the hills of Prescott, Arizona, swinging her arms and savoring the warm, pine-scented air. A prolific letter writer, she spent hours penning exuberant, heartfelt notes to each of her five children. Sad to say, none of this sufficed to combat the isolation, loneliness and hidden factors all beginning to contribute to her declining brain health.

Mom showed signs of confusion as my siblings and I took turns visiting. My four-year-old daughter, Eliza, came along one time. Mom wasn't there to meet us at our prearranged pickup spot, a shopping mall where the bus from the Phoenix airport had dropped us off. During a few sweaty hours on a hot bench, my squirmy child and I made several trips to the pay phone (how inconvenient that cell phones had not yet been invented) and left messages for Mom on her answering machine, to no avail. Finally, I summoned a taxi.

Mom was nonplussed when we arrived. "Oh, you're here," she said. "I thought you were coming tomorrow."

We enjoyed our visit, but I noticed Mom struggling with tasks in the kitchen. Rearranging one of the oven racks frustrated her. While preparing dinner, she appeared stressed and uncertain. I felt sad and worried about what these changes meant for my mother's future.

Not long after that trip, it became clear that Mom should live closer to family. My four siblings and I were spread across the country, but since two of them had settled in Colorado, moving Mom to Denver was the most practical option. Yet considering memory care or assisted living at that point seemed premature. Instead, my brother called on her daily in her senior high-rise, and my sister was also a dedicated visitor, attuned to Mom's every need.

When I heard about Mom's interaction with the security guard, my mind flashed back to when I was in my teens and Grandmother Lois, my father's mother, lived with us for a month or two before entering a nursing home. On my way to the bathroom late one night, I found her awake, wandering in the hallway. I had never before seen her in a nightgown or without her glasses, her silver hair cascading halfway down to her waist instead of being gathered into a tight, sophisticated bun. She resembled a ghost from another era. When she greeted me using the name of one of my sisters, I didn't know how to respond. At that time, I was unaware of the term *dementia*, although I had heard the word *senility*, which I associated with foolishness, madness and inevitable doom.

After Mom's subsequent diagnosis of "probable Alzheimer's disease," I wondered, will Mom become ghostly, like my grandmother? Is she going to forget our names? Might she stop talking altogether? Will she cease to be herself and fade away? I felt a deep emotional bond with my mom, and I couldn't help thinking about whether this might happen to me someday.

Back then, I didn't understand that when Mom felt so lost and alone that she believed taking a taxi ride to Kansas would make everything okay, she was experiencing a normal human response to whatever was happening in her brain. When our present is confusing, stressful or traumatic, who doesn't have moments of tender longing for easier times and familiar places? As is often the case with those who live with dementia, Mom had wandered back in time, thinking herself much younger than her actual age. She and Dad grew up in Junction City. That was where they met as teenagers, fell in love, and became engaged. Mom was very close to her two beloved brothers—one of whom was a fighter pilot whose death shattered her heart when his plane was shot down so close to the end of World War II.

My parents married in California shortly after my father graduated from Stanford in 1936. Mom's caring and protective father, a respected judge, accompanied her on the train for half the journey to California. She was nineteen years old.

"Going home" to the comfort of her family and her past in Junction City made perfect sense to Mom in the middle of that dark, lonesome night on the thirtieth floor. Without her knowledge or consent, her brain was changing abnormally. I find it helpful to remember that regardless of what people living with dementia say, do or think, they are reacting naturally to the mental roadblocks they encounter.

I earned my living in theater for twenty-six years. Looking back, my switch to dementia care makes perfect sense. Both fields require patience, imagination, creativity, trial and error, spontaneity, empathy and practice. Not long after Mom's diagnosis, I was considering my next career direction. Her situation sparked my curiosity and concern, propelled me into dementia care, and ignited a passion to dedicate the rest of my working life to understanding this syndrome and helping those affected by it.

While Alzheimer's is classified as a disease, dementia is not. Instead, it is commonly defined as a clinical syndrome—a collection of symptoms related to a decline in mental functioning that can be caused by many underlying conditions. Each individual living with dementia will show a unique mix of indicators, which makes working in the field complicated—and fascinating.

I am grateful to have learned about dementia from my mother and many others whom geriatrician G. Allen Power identifies as the true experts in dementia: the people who are living with it.

> Over the past several years, I have come to view such people as the "True Experts" in dementia. I do not consider myself an expert; rather, I am a professional student of dementia, and with all due respect to my colleagues in neurology and psychiatry, they are not experts either, because this condition involves a change in our minds and, therefore, in the ways we see, hear and think about the world around us. That is not something the rest of us can completely understand.[1]

1 G. Allen Power, *Dementia Beyond Disease: Enhancing Well-being* (Baltimore, MD: Health Professions Press, 2017 Rev.), 12.

In my experience as a "professional student of dementia," I have been amazed and humbled by the insight, strengths and skills that people living with dementia retain. In memory care communities, a person's deficits too often become the primary focus. The oft-used terms "dementia patient" and "person with dementia" reinforce this by implying an individual is defined by their illness. If I were to receive a dementia diagnosis, I would prefer to be described as someone "living with dementia"—someone who is, above all else, *living* and whose identity extends far beyond a diagnosis. Wouldn't you agree?

Recognizing and utilizing an individual's strengths, interests and talents enhances their well-being. I am inspired by the courage, humor, heart, compassion, creativity and resilience of those living with dementia. Instead of being extinguished by society's typical adverse knee-jerk reaction to this diagnosis, these qualities endure and triumph.

Retained Strengths and Skills of People Living with Dementia

Focusing on the strengths that individuals living with dementia retain will help build relationships, promote engagement, and ensure well-being. These include their:

- sense of humor
- appreciation of music and rhythm
- ability to read nonverbal signals
- long-term memory
- ability to care and express love
- spirit and spirituality
- capacity for gratitude
- interests and passions
- courage and resilience
- creativity

I invite you to meet the growing challenge we face in eldercare: *how to make a dramatic, positive difference for individuals living with dementia*—those we love, live with, live near, care for, or who are otherwise part of our lives and communities.

The Bipartisan Policy Center predicts 4.1 million late baby boomers in the USA will continue to turn sixty-five annually through 2027.[2] As of 2024, the Alzheimer's Association notes that 6.9 million Americans are living with Alzheimer's disease, the most common type of dementia. This number could approach 13 million by 2050 unless medical breakthroughs can prevent, slow or cure the disease.[3] These statistics are indeed daunting, considering Alzheimer's disease is only one of more than a hundred potential causes of dementia.[4]

I wonder: What if everyone who interacts with someone living with dementia—whether in their family, community or workplace—could learn to make life easier for these individuals? Can we look beyond a person's cognitive decline, so living with it doesn't have to feel like the end of a meaningful existence? Can we work to reduce the impact of dementia on those affected, so it doesn't *matter* in such a negative way for the individual?

I don't intend to sound glib or insensitive with these questions. In many respects, dementia is difficult. Without a doubt, it is a profound change that matters a great deal to an individual's health and well-being. Receiving this diagnosis can be an overwhelming shock, presenting complex emotional challenges to individuals and their families. As dementia progresses, the changes can be tough to accept and adapt to for everyone concerned.

---

2 "'Silver tsunami': Record number of Americans set to turn 65 this year," *Axios*, February 19, 2024, emeraldlakebooks.com/silvertsunami.

3 Alzheimer's Association, *2024 Alzheimer's Disease Facts and Figures* (Chicago: Alzheimer's Association, 2024), 21–24, emeraldlakebooks.com/alzheimersfacts.

4 Alzheimer's Disease International, "Types of Dementia," accessed February 22, 2026, emeraldlakebooks.com/dementiatypes.

Caring for someone living with dementia may not be your dream job, whether as a familial obligation or a paid position. As a family member, you may find yourself thrust into the role of care partner without much knowledge about dementia. Finding practical guidance on making life easier, more enjoyable, and more meaningful for your relative might be challenging. An overwhelming mix of fear, grief and frustration about the time and energy caregiving requires can lead to anger. In addition, you may also have financial concerns. To make matters more challenging, if you've had a difficult relationship with a relative who is experiencing dementia, you may feel "stuck" with this new responsibility. Any of these pressures might cause you to think life is nothing but a downhill slide for the individual living with dementia, your relationship with them, and yourself.

If you work in memory care, you may not fully understand what you have signed up for until you've been immersed in your job for a while. Caring for those living with dementia requires considerable time, patience, skill and focus. I have worked with many team members who demonstrate an innate knack for the job, and with others who work hard to develop the requisite skills. Sometimes people struggle and determine that this field is not for them. Employee turnover is a persistent issue, which worsened during the pandemic and resurfaces whenever they determine compensation is insufficient.

I am not suggesting we can just snap our fingers to "make life easier" 24/7 for everyone with this diagnosis. In a secured memory care community, individuals may feel coerced against their will into living in a large, noisy environment that seems far removed from any sense of home. They may have limited interactions with precious loved ones while receiving care from team members who lack the motivation or training to meet the challenges of dementia care with success.

Individuals being taken care of at home may also feel dissatisfied with the limitations of their situation. If they can no longer come and go as they please, if they are no longer permitted to drive, and if all their friends seem to have vanished, home may not feel much like home anymore.

No matter what inspired you to read this book, I promise if you are open to listening to, befriending and learning as much as possible from individuals living with dementia, you will be better equipped to promote their well-being. In addition, you'll discover more minutes or hours—perhaps even days—when dementia doesn't prevent them (or you) from experiencing joy, connection, love, laughter and engagement in the moment.

A Pathway Unfurls

A cause more promising
Than a wild dedication of yourselves
to unpath'd waters, undream'd shores
—William Shakespeare, *The Winter's Tale*, act 4, sc. 4

Mom

When my brother arrives for his early evening visit with Mom at her first memory care residence, he notices she is sitting in front of the TV with other community members and a female aide. They are watching a video.

When he calls to tell me about this later, I think, *Well, at least an aide was with them; maybe she was commenting on the video to keep everyone engaged.* No such luck. My brother explains they were watching a documentary called "Dangerous Dogs."

In lurid, graphic detail, the camera zooms in on the damage, the bloody bites and gashes that vicious canines have inflicted upon individuals of all ages, including young children. Aghast and sickened, and preparing to give management a piece of his furious mind, my brother moves as fast as possible to extricate Mom from the group and away from that screen.

A few weeks later, after a violent incident involving two male members of the community, my siblings secured a new home for Mom in record time.

Mom lived in four different communities during her decade in memory care. Each felt like a small improvement over the last, yet there were always aspects of the care that didn't meet our family's expectations.

When I visited Mom in her second memory care residence, I spent each day with her for most of a week, during which the activities director showed up once, for about forty-five minutes. She handed out paper and pencils. I don't remember what she instructed us to do with these, but I recall feeling like a bona fide resident, doodling with Mom and her companions, all of whom were as bored as I was. Mom, who enjoyed gardening, reading, baking and spending time with children and babies, deserved more stimulating engagement, as did everyone in her community.

The day's mood brightened when Mom introduced me to her new friend, Jocelyn. Before dementia became a barrier for Jocelyn, she worked for many years as an actress in a professional theater company. I was thrilled to learn she had played Rosalind, the lead character in *As You Like It.* Since portraying Gertrude in *Hamlet* (during high school) and Helena in *A Midsummer Night's Dream* (in college), I have been an avowed Shakespeare nut. Jocelyn amazed me by rattling off the "All the world's a stage" speech without hesitation. This well-known passage from *As You Like It* isn't one she would have been required to memorize since Rosalind doesn't speak it. Captivated by Jocelyn's recitation of Shakespeare from her long-term memory, a fuzzy idea began to take shape in my mind.

My first step would be to purchase a trunk on wheels, which would help me bring meaningful, interactive engagement to Mom and her new friends whenever I visited Denver.

I found a helpful resource in *Talking to Alzheimer's* by Claudia J. Strauss, a small, practical, easy read filled with communication-related tips. Published in 2001, this was the first book I ever read about dementia, and it remains useful and relevant today. To learn more, I took a class from the Alzheimer's Association on activity-based care, which emphasized the importance of sensory stimulation for individuals living with dementia.

I went to work adapting my favorite folk tale, *The Fisherman and His Wife*, for my purposes. I searched for and created props that would emerge from my small green trunk into participants' hands to bring the story to life. Strips of colored fabric represented the sea, which changes mood and color multiple times in this magical tale. I planned to have everyone sitting in a circle and to hold one end of each cloth myself while recruiting someone from the group to hold the other. Together, we would raise the fabric up and down to simulate the movement of the waves. When I was ready to debut this activity, I contacted the activities director at Mom's community, who was delighted to put Tales from a Trunk on the schedule during my next visit to Denver.

For another presentation, fun facts about Shakespeare and snippets of scenes offered ample opportunity for audience participation. I dubbed this program Shakespearience. In a playful and reductive take on the balcony scene, I gave myself a workout switching costume pieces to portray Romeo *and* Juliet. It concluded with a rendition of "All the world's a stage," enhanced with various props. When I brought this program to Mom's memory care community, I placed a baby doll in her arms during the line, "First, the infant, mewling and puking in his mother's arms." Mom was pleased to hold the doll (despite the puking reference), and Jocelyn was eager to join me in reciting the speech.

I chose spring-themed poetry for Spring Things and included an adaptation of DuBose Hayward's classic tale *The Country Bunny and the Little Gold Shoes*, in which a mother of twenty-one bunnies is honored to become the Easter Bunny. A Walgreens sale provided all the stuffed baby bunnies needed to tell the story. I handed them out to audience members at the point when Mama Bunny had completed her family. Those tiny, fuzzy bunnies were a huge hit. Several participants clutched three or four at once. I was concerned about getting all twenty-one back at the end, but that turned out not to be an issue.

Seasonal stories from various cultures and A. A. Milne's poem "King John's Christmas" inspired me to develop a fourth program, Holiday Cheer.

Over the next few years, whenever I visited my mom and siblings in Colorado, I brought along my trunk to provide an interactive program for Mom and her community. She enjoyed these sessions, remaining attentive and curious throughout.

It didn't take long to discover I loved interacting with people living with dementia. I started peddling Tales from a Trunk for a modest fee to memory care communities in the Minneapolis area, and others in and around Denver. Although I was having a lot of fun, attempting to support myself this way was discouraging. I decided to search for an activities coordinator position where I could focus on working with these individuals.

My first two job interviews led nowhere, but at the third one, the campus administrator was intrigued by the idea of someone with a theater background serving as the activities coordinator for those in memory care. At St. Therese Southwest, now known as The Glenn Hopkins, my starting salary was a humbling $12.15 per hour (I was fifty years old). However, the education I received over the twelve years I worked there proved invaluable. In time, I persuaded St. Therese to create the position of memory care coordinator, which I held while earning my master's degree in gerontology. Both experiences equipped me well for my eventual role as dementia program coordinator for Ebenezer Management Services, where I was responsible for establishing best practices and training others in dementia care across multiple sites.

St. Therese Southwest had been an independent senior housing complex known as The Towers for many years. My job began one week before the opening of our new assisted living building, The Terraces, which was connected to The Towers by a long hallway and included a secured twelve-person memory care floor.

As individuals moved in, I had the luxury of getting to know them one at a time. We opened the second floor of our memory care residence a few years later, adding eighteen additional apartments. My job responsibilities expanded, but this gave me the opportunity to meet, care for, and learn from many more individuals. Most of the stories I'll share to illustrate what I have learned about dementia and dementia care come from the years I spent in regular contact with these people.

Once I'd gotten my feet wet in the realm of dementia care, I noticed several acquaintances reacted with alarm when, after they asked what I was doing for work now, I replied, "I work with people who have dementia."

"Oh!" they gasped, shuddering. "That must be so depressing!"

"Actually," I countered, "it's more fun than I've ever had."

That was only a slight exaggeration. I adored my actor friends and took pride in my involvement in theater. However, working with individuals living with dementia turned out to be more stimulating and fulfilling. The job requirements felt more in sync with what I had to offer. I could use skills from my theater training with a sense of freedom and confidence I'd rarely experienced on stage. The stakes were higher.

I had to be present to do my best for the human beings in front of me. My work wasn't about my performance or feeling good enough; this was about them and the significant needs they couldn't manage for themselves. Theater helped cultivate the curiosity, creativity and empathy needed to integrate the lessons I was learning from daily interactions with people experiencing abnormal brain changes.

I don't mean to imply a theater background is the only viable springboard into dementia care. Rest assured that any tools or experiences that have enabled you to make authentic connections, build strong relationships, show compassion for others, express joy, or be creative will translate well into making a significant, positive difference for these individuals.

Now, allow me to introduce you to my teachers and the lessons they imparted to me. Some were exceptional educators—and you'll see them multiple times.

Connecting First

Promise me friendship

—William Shakespeare, *Timon of Athens*, act 4, sc. 3

Mona

Mona is tall, gaunt and miserable. I must say, she is the surliest resident of our memory care community. Her usual mood is a blend of sour regret and disgust. It's rare to see family visit her. She is challenging to communicate with for many team members, including me. Her favorite resident assistant, Becky, has earned her trust, but others struggle to keep her on an even keel.

As the activities coordinator for memory care, I oversee snack time. Today, Mona and Becky arrive early and take a seat. As I walk over to their table, I focus on making my voice as sunny as possible. "Would you like coffee or lemonade?" Mona shoots me a glare of disdainful irritation and responds to my overly sing-song approach with three words: "Just. Say. Hi."

> If we don't connect before diving into a chore, we have a slim chance of building trust.

Yikes, did Mona ever put me in my rightful place! Despite my Tales from a Trunk experience, I was clueless about the importance of the first few seconds of interaction when performing a task for a person who is living with dementia. If we don't connect before diving into a chore, we have a slim chance of building trust, the foundation of a good relationship, and we miss the opportunity to make a meaningful, dramatic difference for that person. Even though I was embarrassed, I vowed to do better.

> I take a breath. Lowering the tone of my voice to a more natural level, I sit down at their table and say, "Hello, Mona. Hi, Becky." We chat for a while before I deliver their beverages and snacks.

Looking back, I regret not adding, "I'm glad you're here." I still had a lot to learn. Even though I didn't have the presence of mind to thank Mona for her reprimand, better late than never... Thank you, Mona, for reminding me to greet people by name, shake their hands if that's their preference, and do my best to make them feel welcome, safe and seen before diving into my agenda.

Though Mona lived with dementia, she was perceptive enough to recognize that I had not taken the time to *see* her. No wonder this aroused exasperation and anger. Maya Angelou popularized the saying, "People will forget what you said, people will forget what you did, but people will never forget how you made them feel."[5] I have found this true of all human beings, including

5 Garson O'Toole, "People Will Forget What You Said, People Will Forget What You Did, but People Will Never Forget How You Made Them Feel," Quote Investigator, April 6, 2014, emeraldlakebooks.com/mayaangelou.

those who experience dementia. When interacting with such individuals, considering how you want them to *feel* is helpful.

In residential care communities, a key practice for building relationships is for care team members to acknowledge individuals while passing in the hallway. Smiling at people, waving to them, and greeting them by name are effective ways to connect and say, "I'm glad to see you." How often do elders feel genuinely seen by others? Suppose we rush through a corridor to move from point A to point B, ignoring everyone we pass who might appreciate a smile, a wave or a hello. The result is a missed opportunity to make a significant difference in how those in our care experience their environment (which many community marketing materials promote as, *ahem*, "home-like").

Anyone who insists they "don't have time" to connect because of all the items on their ever-demanding to-do list should consider the advice of occupational therapist and dementia care specialist Teepa Snow, who often says, in her training, "You don't have time *not* to do it!"[6] I have heard other dementia trainers and practitioners echo this idea. Consider how long it can take when you must deal with an individual who feels so alone, bored or desperate for compassion and meaningful human connection that they decide to punch someone, scream, pack up all their belongings to go home, or try to find a way out of the prison of your secured building.

One morning, I learned that Charlie, a sweet man who had moved in a few days earlier and was at risk for falls, had escaped the night before through a first-floor window. We were relieved, grateful and lucky he was found a few frantic hours after his departure, unharmed, at an apartment building down the street. That incident could have had tragic consequences. Aside from

6 Teepa Snow and Positive Approach to Care (PAC), presentation at the Minnesota History Center, Saint Paul, Minnesota. November 12, 2019.

ensuring windows in our senior communities are secure, we must dedicate the necessary time to connect with, comfort and build trust with those living with dementia as if their lives depended on it—because they very well might.

Putting It Into Practice

To prepare yourself to connect with an individual in your care:

1. Feel your feet on the ground as you walk.
2. Take a few deep breaths.
3. Relax your eyes and the rest of your face.
4. Pause and remind yourself of what you know about this individual or what you would like to learn about them.
5. Calmly approach them with curiosity and a smile on your face.
6. Be open to being guided by the person.
7. Think: *This could be fun.*

Connecting first and building relationships with those in our care helps us better understand what it might feel like inside their heads.

Living with an Uncooperative Brain

How are our brains beguiled
—William Shakespeare, *Sonnets*, No. 59

Evelyn

"I feel like I have to meet the train, but I don't know what the schedule is." Out of the blue, Evelyn confides this to me one day as we pass in the hallway.

She reminds me of a hothouse flower whose bloom will be destroyed if the temperature, soundscape and humidity aren't calibrated to perfection. On the other side of her fragility, Evelyn is a trouper, a good sport with a healthy sense of humor. Still, her sunny moods can flip into nerves, morph into anxiety, and escalate into full-fledged agitation.

Evelyn loves the color purple. Today, she sports purple pants, a long-sleeved purple velveteen top, and her trademark gray felt hat.

Her tone is resigned yet frustrated when she refers to the train she feels she must meet. Though she is well past the point of being aware of her Alzheimer's diagnosis, Evelyn is full of insight into what living with dementia is like. When she mentions having to meet the train, her intended meaning hovers like a cloud, halfway between the literal and the symbolic. Part of her understands she has no train to catch; what she's missing is something else. The other part believes she needs to be somewhere she is not. If only she could recall where that place is, how to get there, and where in the world she put the car keys. Moreover, now that she thinks about it, she can't for the life of her remember where she parked…

Another day, after breakfast, Evelyn is having a tough morning. I've seldom seen her struggle this much to put a sentence together. Unable to decipher her garbled speech, I'm on the verge of taking her to see the nurse when the word *bathroom* emerges from a sudden outpouring of nonsensical syllables. I offer to show her to the nearest restroom down the hall. Evelyn nods and trudges along, chewing her bottom lip and concentrating on maneuvering her walker. Her face contorts like a student trying to pick the correct answer on an exam.

I hold the restroom door open and follow her in. Though she can manage on her own, I stick around in case she needs extra help today. I lock the door and move into a corner of the small bathroom. Evelyn stops short a few feet away from the toilet, her gaze riveted on the floor.

Without looking my way, she proclaims with surprising energy, "This floor! It looks just like my brain."

Her speech is clear as a bell. I inspect the grayish-green floor to see what she might mean. It's covered with two-inch square tiles and is dustier than one would prefer, but apart from that

> there's nothing of note. Every part of it looks like every other part. Boring. No direction, nothing of interest. Dull, dull, dull.

Later that day, I returned to the bathroom. I couldn't get Evelyn's comment out of my head. I took a photo of the floor tiles and showed it to my husband, Phil, that evening. His response was, "Huh. It's like a crossword puzzle without any clues."

What a valuable glimpse into the current backdrop of her mind Evelyn had offered that morning. Her remark taught me that we must work to transform what I suspect many people living with dementia experience far too often: a landscape filled with emptiness, suffused with boredom; a stage setting full of dead ends and roadblocks; an overwhelming sense of dread, of being lost in a puzzle with no clue how to escape. Doubtless, dementia *mattered* to Evelyn that morning—in a dark, dusty, distressing way.

There is a gift in accepting the challenges that people living with dementia may present.

I realized I needed to expand my understanding, to consider what reality feels like for these individuals. It's easy but unfair to blame them for being difficult and making our jobs challenging to the point of discomfort. Isn't their chore of dealing with an uncooperative brain tougher than ours?

I learned from Evelyn and many others that there is a gift in accepting the challenges that people living with dementia may present. A door swings open, inviting us to explore, empathize and understand that each individual is doing their absolute best given the changes occurring in their brain. We begin to imagine what might be beneficial for them. When our chosen strategy proves effective, we incorporate that tool into our ever-evolving toolbox. Of course, not every tactic works for everyone all the time. That's why we need a substantial toolkit to handle the various situations and emotions that may arise. We expand it and increase our confidence with each person we are privileged to know, care for, and learn from.

The more I understood what dementia felt like for Evelyn, the easier it became to build trust with her, empathize with her concerns, and ensure our interactions were positive and helpful.

I discovered she delighted in gazing at and discussing the glamorous black-and-white photo of herself in her 1950s wedding dress, displayed in the shadow box outside her apartment door. She was excited to show me the framed picture on her dresser of herself standing alongside "The King of Golf," Arnold Palmer, with their golf bags.

As I learned about the memories that had meant so much to Evelyn, I added mini-golf to the schedule. I also planned a Wedding Reminisce activity featuring a 1950s pearl-encrusted satin wedding dress that had belonged to the mother of a dear friend of mine. Our ladies loved touching the fabric, smoothing its wrinkles, and reminiscing about what they had worn at their weddings. Several who had married during the war discussed how they'd had to forgo fancy gowns in favor of simple suits. Since Evelyn and many other women in our community adored hats and scarves, I set up a display in our activity room with items for them to admire, try on, and, yes, on occasion, "take home." (I simply retrieved them later, when I knew people were not in their apartments.)

To attract more men to activities, I invited Peter, a volunteer from The Towers, to showcase his prized collection of miniature classic cars. He talked about each replica in turn and passed them around the circle. Both men and women enjoyed handling them and reminiscing about their favorite vehicles. A reclusive gentleman named Ben ventured out of his apartment for the first time to attend this activity.

When we provide engagement and interactions that match the specific interests and hobbies of individuals in our care, we validate their passions, remind them of their skills and accomplishments, and offer a detour around the stumbling blocks and puzzles affecting their brains.

Providing opportunities for individuals to share experiences and favorite pastimes with peers (and caregivers) fosters meaningful relationships.

Relationships with Caregivers

I count myself in nothing else so happy
As in a soul remembering my good friends

—William Shakespeare, *Richard II*, act 2, sc. 3

Evelyn

After unlocking my postage-stamp-sized office, I barely have time to sit before Lila, one of our dining room servers, appears in my doorway. Instead of her usual smile, her brow is furrowed as she pleads with me to help Evelyn, who is lingering at her table long after breakfast.

"She says she's going to pass out," Lila says worriedly.

I grab my radio, thinking I might need to contact a nurse. (*Is there one on site today? It's a holiday.*) I'm grateful my office is close to the dining room.

When I enter, Evelyn is pushing her walker with weary determination on the far side of the room and looking pale. As I draw nearer, I notice she's more hunched than usual.

"Hi, Evelyn. What's going on?"

Evelyn stops walking. "I just don't have any pep."

These days, Evelyn alternates between crystal-clear statements like that one and others so peppered with substitutions that you have to listen for the emotion behind her words to grasp what she's trying to convey.

"Would you like to lie down?"

"Yes, I think so."

We trudge down the long hallway to her studio apartment.

When we get there, she plops down on her single bed with a heavy sigh. After a serious discussion about the relative merits of taking her shoes off or keeping them on, I help her get her feet up on the bed. She decides to keep her shoes on to be "ready to go" later. I approve of her choice, cover her with a light blanket, smooth her forehead, and give her a soft kiss on the cheek.

"You know something?" she asks in her familiar, quavering voice. "You're my freezie, and I just love my freezie!"

Evelyn's meaning was unmistakable. She'd told me I was her friend. I even noticed that, if you rotate the "z" in "freezie" forty-five degrees to form an "n," it appears Evelyn incorporated all but one of the letters from the word "friend" into her invented word.

If I asked you to list three things that make your life meaningful—things you could not bear to live without—I bet you would include "family" or "friends" on that list, or at least the name of one person who is special to you. Dr. John Brose, a leading national authority on aging and behavioral health, asserts "the quality of life for individuals living with dementia depends on the quality of the relationships they have" with the people they spend the most time with.[7] This insight holds true for all of us. Relationships that nurture us are vital for our well-being.

In a memory care or skilled nursing setting, if you're a resident assistant, certified nursing assistant, therapeutic recreation director, or activities coordinator, chances are you interact more with a person living with dementia than their family members do. I'm positive you spend more time with them than any of their visiting friends do, if indeed your community members are fortunate enough to have any who visit. However, you might not feel an easy connection with every person in your care or with those you support in daily activities. Or, as a family member caring for someone with dementia, you may not have had a close relationship with this relative.

Developing rapport and mutual trust with those living with dementia is crucial for their overall well-being.

Developing rapport and mutual trust with those living with dementia is crucial for their overall well-being , but engaging with people we don't know, haven't met before, or feel little connection with can be intimidating. We may wonder if (or how) we can gain their trust. If we are patient and willing to learn more about them, the relationship will shift, allowing us to view the individual in a new light. We may uncover a sense of humor behind their grumpy complaints or start to empathize with the loneliness beneath their defensive exterior. If we become more open and accepting of who a person is, this allows them to guide us in how best to connect with them. Once a pathway to a relationship emerges, our tasks become easier and more enjoyable.

When we work in residential care, the relationships we develop will not feel the same as those we have with our closest loved ones,

7 John Brose, "Challenging Situations: The New Customer," presentation at Martin Luther Campus, Bloomington, Minnesota, August 23, 2016.

nor should they. There are personal boundaries that healthcare workers are mandated to respect and must not cross. While the connections we form with the people we serve differ from those with our dearest friends and family, they are valuable and can be filled with genuine affection. They are not about pretending. As relationships with those in our care evolve, we share laughter, become curious about their lives, and enjoy a sense of ease when we are around them. In the process, we learn to communicate that we understand their concerns and support their interests. We discover how to encourage them when they are struggling.

You may notice all this sounds a lot like how we interact with our closest friends. In fact, David Troxel and Virginia Bell, authors of *The Best Friends Approach to Alzheimer's Care* and companion books, have made precisely this comparison for years when promoting the concept of excellence in dementia care.

Jane and Amahle

I'm in the middle of throwing a birthday party for Jane. Five ladies who live on her floor are seated with us around the table. Soon, we'll sing "Happy Birthday," and I'll divvy up the angel food cake.

Jane, a hearty, independent woman with a lilting voice, sits at the head of the table. I marvel at her joyful, confident presence while she shares memories of working at a university and singing in multiple choirs over the years.

As we chat, Amahle, a regular resident assistant on this floor, appears in the open doorway of the activity room. Calm, gentle and wise, she is three decades older than most of our resident assistants.

Seeing Amahle, Jane flutters her hands in excitement. "Oh, oh! Come in, come in! You must stay for cake!"

> Amahle enters and wraps Jane in a hug, after which Jane introduces her to everyone as if none of us had ever met her. She describes Amahle as the "kindest, most helpful, most wonderful person" she has known. In this moment, it feels like the party is for Amahle, and Jane is giving an eloquent speech in her honor.

Jane's testimonial offers a powerful lesson about the profound impact of a strong, meaningful relationship between a caregiver and an individual living with dementia. Amahle was a natural at earning trust and learning the details of what a person needed from her. She was originally from Kenya, where it is common for elders to continue living with their families. One time, Yusuf, Amahle's husband (another stellar care attendant), assured me, "We care for these people as though they are our family." I do not doubt that many in our community benefited from the sincerity of Amahle and Yusuf's commitment to building authentic relationships.

As Brose says, "The most powerful medication we have is not in the med carts. It's us, the way we interact with the people in our care."[8]

8 John Brose, "Challenging Situations: The New Customer."

Sustaining a Meaningful Marriage

I am half yourself
—William Shakespeare, *The Merchant of Venice*, act 3, sc. 2

Meg and Will

"I think Alzheimer's is worse than death."

Will blurts this out at the beginning of our care partner support group meeting, which I facilitate. Will's wife, Meg, has lived in our memory care community for about six months.

It's a chilling moment. I'm shocked, but my role is to support discussion around the concerns and feelings of the group members, not to challenge any opinions expressed.

"It can be tough to witness the decline," I reply, stifling the argument I am tempted to start—that Meg still has many strengths and is such a delightful person.

Meg grew up in Brooklyn, New York, singing at the piano alongside her mother, an accomplished piano teacher, while I grew up in Ridgewood, New Jersey, half an hour away. Meg and I also share a fondness for Broadway show tunes. Walking down the hallway together, we often sing "Getting to Know You" from *The King and I.* She knows the lyrics to the verses better than I do, and she sings better too.

Meg lives with vascular dementia, which can include emotional highs and lows, and occasionally, she is overwhelmed with sadness and tears. Will's comment stemmed from legitimate grief, reflecting an acute and profound loss he felt more than I could imagine at that point. I could have done better to validate his feelings. Of course, he longed to pull Meg back to where her cognition had been before—to turn back time to before dementia interfered.

More often than not, the Meg I knew was vibrant, intelligent and energetic. At Will's insistence, they would walk around our building complex during his daily visits. Their routine included climbing up and down several long flights of stairs. (This was decades before exercise was widely recognized as one of the best things you can do for your brain.) Despite Will's pessimistic comment during the group meeting, he did all he could to maintain his wife's health and keep their relationship alive. His actions spoke louder than his words, demonstrating that their marriage remained meaningful to him.

Years later, I can well relate to the dread of a disease that causes a loved one's decline. My husband, Phil, died at age sixty-one from metastatic melanoma. This cancer presented as a brain tumor, diagnosed two years to the day before he slipped away from this life. An accomplished theater professional, his timing was always impeccable.

Phil was proud of his mind, which he used to best advantage when acting, directing and writing. He was brilliant and hilarious in unique ways. Often, the very first thing he said in the morning made me laugh. I still wonder how he did that.

During his illness, Phil underwent two different types of radiation treatments: gamma knife, which precisely targets the tumor site, and whole-brain, which treats the entire brain to reduce the risk of additional tumor growth. He experienced severe side effects, including a burst colon, which required emergency surgery in the middle of one traumatic night.

Later, while receiving hospice care at home, Phil transformed into a much older version of himself. He became way too thin. He no longer chattered with his trademark enthusiasm. His inimitable sense of humor was less pronounced.

> In the middle of the night, Phil gets out of bed to use the bathroom. I follow behind because he's walking with his torso parallel to the floor. I'm scared he might fall.
>
> "What are you doing? Get away from me!" he snaps, sensing my proximity and panic.
>
> This irritability is uncharacteristic. Stunned, I back off but hover as close as I dare.
>
> He's acting not unlike someone who is living with dementia. I try to pretend I didn't have that thought, but I cannot deny Phil's unusual posture and emotional state are related to a "progressive decline in mental functioning," a phrase often used to define dementia. I realize this experience must be similar to what many people face when caring for someone living with dementia at home.

Was it, in fact, dementia I witnessed that night? Who knows? Did it matter, given Phil's situation?

Professor and researcher Antonio E. Damin and his colleagues have determined radiation (a.k.a. radiotherapy) delivered to the brain can cause symptoms of dementia.[9] (I didn't think to look that up until writing this narrative.)

After that night, I had to accept I couldn't bring Phil back to where I wanted him to be. I couldn't expect him to interact with me like he had before. This journey was his, and it was heading in an unchangeable direction. He had no choice but to follow. As his care partner, wife and longtime best friend, my role was to respect and support him wherever he was during this time.

Phil's decline from that point was gentle, sweet and sometimes funny. One afternoon, Eliza, his devoted twenty-six-year-old stepdaughter, whom he nicknamed "Lizard" when she was twelve, was chatting with him on his hospital bed in the living room.

"We have a *lot* of pants," Phil remarks.

Eliza's eyes widen as a bemused half-smile spreads across her face.

He elaborates. "But my sister and brother-in-law have *even more* pants than we do."

She follows his gaze to the tall bookcase standing at the end of his bed. "You mean books?"

"No! *Pants!*"

Eliza has no choice but to giggle.

"Pants" is a funny word, as I remember Phil pointed out before his cancer diagnosis, perhaps during dinner while educating us on the finer points of comedy.

Time passed. Phil grew quieter—strange for an actor and comic genius who delighted in projecting his voice to the rafters,

9 Antonio E. Damin et al., "Dementia Post-radiotherapy: Improvement with Acetylcholinesterase Inhibitor. A Case Report." Dementia & Neuropsychologia 3, no. 1 (2009): 68–72, doi.org/10.1590/S1980-57642009DN30100013.

even in our small, rafter-less house. Eliza and I felt privileged to be by his side at the threshold of his transition. We learned to trust that his essence was still there. Love bound us, no matter what. Phil still cared for us and would remain part of us forever.

The Ability to Care and to Love

They are so link'd in friendship
—William Shakespeare, *III Henry VI*, act 4, sc. 1

Ruby and Janet

Ruby's nonsensical speech is as bubbly as champagne. She is a tall, vibrant woman with sky-blue eyes and stylish chin-length silver hair. Often speaking in complete gibberish, Ruby's exuberant tone suggests she means, "Isn't that the most amazing thing you've ever seen?"

Since people who speak in gibberish tend to understand your speech without a problem, I respond using a similar tone. "Oh, yes, Ruby, I agree. That is wonderful!"

Janet presents a stark contrast to Ruby. Small in stature, with thin, tousled gray hair, her voice is always a hoarse whisper.

It's a quiet, sunny afternoon, just after lunch, and most of our community members have returned to their apartments for a rest. From the hallway, I notice Ruby and Janet are the only people in the activity room. Curious to observe how they communicate and what they are up to, I join them.

Janet is standing and cradling a baby doll as though she's holding the most precious being in the world. As she whispers sweet nothings while gazing into the baby's eyes, her head moves ever so slightly from side to side. I remember whispering to Eliza that way when she was an infant.

Ruby watches, silent and entranced as I sit down next to her. She flashes me a grin before returning her eager gaze to Janet and her baby. A minute passes in peaceful silence before Ruby turns to me once more. With perfect clarity, she proclaims, "She has the most beautiful mother!"

This poignant scene was full of lessons. I witnessed a testament to the indomitable spirits of both Ruby and Janet, their ability to care for others and to express affection, and the significance of relationships, regardless of dementia-related communication challenges. Ruby's admiration for Janet and her sheer delight in that moment were powerful enough to silence her gibberish for a while. Janet's laser-focused whispers to her "baby" resonated with affectionate wonder.

Dementia trainer and consultant Megan Carnarius asserts "the heart remains intact"[10] for a person living with dementia. Ruby and Janet provided evidence to support Megan's insight, along with the profound realization that the depth of our humanity is connected to our hearts and spirits, not dependent on our brain function. Though some individuals living with dementia may not offer proof as clearly as Ruby and Janet, I recommend we

10 Megan Carnarius, "A Deeper Perspective on Alzheimer's and Other Dementias," presentation at the Contemplative Caregiver Retreat, Natural Dharma Fellowship, Wonderwell Mountain Refuge, Springfield, New Hampshire, November 13, 2022.

trust Megan's wisdom and look deeply into the humanity and hearts of those living with dementia.

Meg and Evelyn

Two women appear, arm in arm, in the doorway to my tiny office. Meg wears an olive-green sweater, a color not everyone can pull off. With her pale skin, dark hair, and deep blue eyes, Meg qualifies. As usual, Evelyn sports a hat—a stylish purple one today-with a flowery scarf. The effect is classy, despite a stain on her blouse and several mismatched buttons.

As though arriving at a tea party, Evelyn sweeps her arm toward her beloved companion and announces with cheerful pride, "This is my son-in-law!"

Meg responds with an eye roll and an embarrassed laugh, but she's a good sport. With a fond sigh in Evelyn's direction, she gushes back, "This is my little sweetheart!"

At the moment, Meg believes Evelyn is her granddaughter. Tomorrow, she might think Evelyn is her daughter. Evelyn takes today's endearment in stride as she often does (unless she's not in the mood, thank you very much), just as Meg accepts Evelyn's confusion. Today, all is gleeful and festive. Anything goes.

This pageant in my doorway is delightful and amusing. The display of affection these two exchange is sweet, touching and genuine. It is heartwarming to see their connection defy the confusion on both sides, meet in the middle, and have a party.

Meg and Evelyn confirmed my belief that relationships between people living with dementia are not only possible, but essential. They showed me how soothing these friendships can be, despite cognitive challenges. Humans often gravitate toward others who share circumstances and are of a similar age. Friendships may blossom between individuals because they are dining room companions or neighbors on the same floor, or because they happened to sit together at an activity. I've known people in memory care who refuse to attend an event unless their special buddy is guaranteed to be there too. Many times, individuals are drawn into activities once they see their friend is already there or because that individual encourages them to join the fun.

Likewise, friendships between people living with dementia and those who volunteer to assist them may develop through various pathways.

Fostering Friendships

I will befriend thee

—William Shakespeare, *Titus Andronicus*, act 3, sc. 1

Friends Indeed

On the first night of my graduate school program, my Social Gerontology professor showed a documentary about elders in Japan who had fled the homes of their sons and daughters. As more Japanese women joined the workforce during the late 1990s, no one was available at home to interact with and care for older family members. The video focused on elders who flocked to a local bathhouse out of a longing for community. The place was open 24/7. Each person received a bowl of rice for lunch and a thin mat to sleep on in the large community room. A few belongings could fit into the tall, skinny locker assigned to each person.

One scene in the video seared itself into my memory:

> A wistful older woman, folding up her sweater with care and stowing it in her locker, tells the camera, "I just want to be of use."

Loneliness is a painful plague for elders, particularly for those living with dementia who lack social interaction and opportunities to make a difference in the lives of others. The woman who "just wanted to be of use" inspired me to focus my thesis project on volunteerism and older adults. After researching related studies, I designed and implemented a program to recruit and train volunteers from The Towers. The dual focus for my Friends InDeed volunteers was to befriend people in our memory care community and to assist with activities.

Loneliness is a painful plague for elders, particularly for those living with dementia.

Sometimes, we gain insight into connecting with someone living with dementia by observing those who do so with ease.

Roger and Pam

Roger will never act on suggestions from others until he feels good and ready to do so, which can take a while. An Army veteran, he is a quiet, tenacious, independent guy with a wry, offbeat sense of humor. Since moving in several months ago, none of our resident assistants have been able to convince him to let them trim his extra-long, creepy fingernails.

Pleasant, chatty and fun-loving, Pam is an energetic bundle of goodwill. Her volunteer assignment includes helping with manicures for the women in our memory care community. As luck would have it, Roger is sitting near the manicure corner in our activity room today.

I whisper to Pam, who is finishing up with Evelyn. "I don't know if Roger will let you get near his nails, but you can try. He needs a major trim."

> Pam goes to Roger, checks his hands, and declares with authority, "Roger, we're going to do your nails now. That's all there is to it. You need a manicure."
>
> Lo and behold, there is no pushback. Roger allows Pam to trim his extra-long nails.

A few months later, Roger became resistant to care. He was overdue for a shower, and the resident assistants were frustrated that their approaches with him were ineffective. Nursing brought in Brent Clairmont, a psychiatric nurse, to evaluate Roger and advise the team. Brent visited with him to learn about his family, and I informed Brent about Pam's success with Roger's nails.

Brent's guidance for our care team aligned with Pam's initial instinct when meeting Roger—he needs a firm, no-nonsense approach. If your approach is meek, Brent explained, he is apt to bulldoze over you with a refusal, but if you use a firm approach, there's a greater chance he'll accept your plan.

Brent pointed out that in addition to Pam's no-nonsense attitude, her proximity in age to Roger helped gain his trust and friendship. Roger grew up surrounded by three strong, influential women: his mother, grandmother and sister. Brent reasoned that to establish a productive relationship with him, one must behave more like the women Roger admired and felt close to.

June and Alice

> June and Alice were fast friends and next-door neighbors six years earlier at The Towers. Their friendship was put on hold when June and her husband, Wally, moved to The Terraces Assisted Living because of his health issues. Wally passed away a few months ago, and now June has transitioned to our memory care residence.

During recruitment for Friends InDeed, Alice, a steadfast, down-to-earth sort, is reluctant to commit. She has reservations due to concerns about her own declining cognition, but once she learns she could become a frequent visitor for her old friend, June, she changes her tune.

When June opens her door to us on Alice's first visit, June's jaw drops at the sight of her former neighbor. They hug and squeal like excited teenagers before June ushers us into her apartment. We settle into a cozy corner for an enthusiastic chat for forty-five minutes, the allotted time for today. Back in the hallway, Alice and June hug each other goodbye, embrace once more, and kiss each other's cheeks, still marveling at the joy of their reunion.

Despite June's dementia, she well remembered the next-door neighbor she had missed for far too long. Alice enjoyed volunteering to help with other activities, but her regular visits with June continued to be her favorite.

People often hesitate to maintain friendships with individuals diagnosed with dementia. If you lack access to information about what to expect or advice on interacting with those diagnosed, you might feel uncomfortable continuing a relationship. You may assume your friend has forgotten you, thinking, "What's the use of trying to connect?"

If your friend lives in an assisted living or skilled care community, you could consult with an activities team member, therapeutic recreation director, nurse or memory care coordinator for suggestions on how to connect. Should you have time, you might explore volunteer opportunities at the site. Often, volunteers in memory care receive training on how to interact with individuals living with dementia. If your friend still lives at home, their care partner may have valuable tips and insights to share with you.

Regardless of where your friend resides, modifying a favorite pastime you used to enjoy together can nurture your relationship. This may involve trial and error, brainstorming and seeking advice from others. When Evelyn moved into our memory care residence, she no longer played golf, although she enjoyed our regular mini-golf activity. I bet she would have loved having one of her former golf buddies take her to the course for lunch at the clubhouse on a beautiful, sunny day.

Research Related to Volunteering

Philip A. Rozario established that older adults who volunteered reported higher levels of well-being, energy, self-esteem and self-confidence, and had lower rates of depression, stress and mortality.[11]

Nancy Morrow-Howell et al. found that while about 100 hours per year (or 2–3 hours per week) provided the maximum benefit, even low levels of volunteering led to positive outcomes.[12]

Since 1986, David Snowdon has followed a group of 678 Catholic sisters in the Nun Study. His research suggests people who pursue their dreams, have a deep sense of spirituality, and are connected to community are more likely to be spared the effects of heart disease

---

11 Rozario, Philip A. "Volunteering Among Current Cohorts of Older Adults and Baby Boomers." *Generations: Journal of the American Society on Aging* 30, no. 4 (2006): 31–6. jstor.org/stable/26555475.

12 Nancy Morrow-Howell, James Hinterlong, Philip A. Rozario and Fengyan Tang, "Effects of Volunteering on the Well-Being of Older Adults," *Journal of Gerontology: Psychological Sciences and Social Sciences* 58, no. 3 (May 2003): S137–45, doi.org/10.1093/geronb/58.3.s137.

and stroke, both of which can increase one's chances of developing dementia.[13]

Belinda and Ethel

If you were in the hallway of The Willows, our second-floor memory care community, and overheard Belinda speaking, you might have assumed she was a twelve- or thirteen-year-old girl visiting a grandparent. Along with her youthful voice, Belinda, in her mid-seventies, was well known in our residence for her gentle heart and sunny disposition.

During an initial focus group meeting to ask potential volunteers what questions they had about dementia, Ethel, a thoughtful, devout Catholic, wondered how she could ever develop a friendship with someone who lives with significant memory loss. Once I assured her she would receive volunteer training, she signed up to help with our Walking Club.

During their strolls, Ethel and Belinda developed a special connection. Following a walk one morning, Ethel escorted Belinda into the activity room for seated exercise. I overheard Belinda say, "Thank you for your help." Without missing a beat, Ethel replied, "Thank you for your friendship."

At our Friends InDeed check-in meeting, Ethel announces that after volunteering for a month, she is happy to continue. "That Belinda is so friendly and loving. I could just hug her every day. She walks better than I can. When a few of us were separated during Walking Club and had to take a different elevator, Belinda was concerned about *me*. She took my hand when I exited the elevator and led me to the window. And I

13 David Snowden, *Aging with Grace* (New York: Bantam Books, 2021), 186–94.

told myself, my God, there's nothing wrong with her! I think it's all about giving them that direct eye contact to say: You're great. You've done a great job."

Dottie and Anne

Anne is another volunteer who, in her late 70s, appears younger than one might expect. Mindful of her own unsteady feet, she uses a walker for safety. Her compassion for those in memory care is evident.

Today, I'm the bingo caller. By popular demand, it remains a staple on our calendar. I appreciate the opportunity it provides for volunteers to bond with those they assist.

Dottie, whom Anne helps on a regular basis, has not yet arrived. A worried expression settles onto Anne's face. "Is Dottie at the beauty shop today?"

"No," I say, explaining Dottie's daughter-in-law washes Dottie's long, silver hair once a week.

Anne smiles. "Dottie reminds me of my grandmother because of her hair, along with the crinkles around her eyes and the way she laughs so hard but tries to stifle it at the same time."

Dottie has macular degeneration, like Anne's grandmother, and she needs help to find the bingo numbers, despite her supersized card.

It's time to begin the game. "Welcome to bingo, everyone," I announce into the karaoke microphone. "Be sure to cover your free space."

Anne sighs. "I guess Dottie's not feeling up to it today. I'll help Betsy, although she doesn't really seem to need it."

After a few numbers are called, in comes Dottie, pushing her walker. She's a big presence, a high-spirited woman prone to calling out "Whoo-hoo!" at the top of her lungs if she needs anything. She hasn't seen Anne yet, but Anne sees her and is already pushing away the empty chair beside her to give Dottie enough room to position her walker, which she prefers to sit on.

I leave my post to guide Dottie as she "lowers the boom," as she enjoys saying.

Relieved after a successful landing, Dottie's eyes settle on Anne and her face lights up like someone has switched on the holiday display in a storefront window. Loud enough for the entire room to hear, she cries out, "Oh, there's my friend, my helper!"

Anne is beaming, and I am too.

The interactions between Friends InDeed participants and those they befriended illustrate numerous ways in which genuine attachments may form between individuals living with dementia and volunteers. The same reasons that bring together people who don't live with dementia are at play. A connection may start by noticing an attitude or a way of being that you respect or resonate with, a friendship rekindled, sincere gratitude for someone's help, a common sense of humor, or being reminded of a beloved relative. Relationships can flourish from simple goodwill and kind intentions on both sides.

When the bonds of friendship are strong, we have an easier time smoothing the way for those who are living with dementia.

Smoothing the Way

How well my comfort is revived by this!
—William Shakespeare, *Romeo and Juliet*, act 3, sc. 3

Janet

Janet reminds me a little of the cartoon character Olive Oyl. I'm not sure why. Perhaps it's her dark, calf-length skirts and her petite, slender frame. Her style is simple even though she spent years selling women's clothing at a major downtown department store.

Janet's personality, however, is a sharp contrast to Popeye's shrill, gangly girlfriend. She is calm, loving and agreeable. Whenever I smile and reach out my hand, she takes it and comes along.

In the six or seven years I've worked with Janet, I've never known a family member to visit her—until today. I have been informed that Janet's daughter, son and daughter-in-law are now waiting in the lobby, asking to see her. So I take her out to join them.

Though Janet's family members greet her with smiles and hugs, she appears confused and overwhelmed.

Her son Tim has flown in from another state and hasn't seen her for a long time. "Hey, Mom, guess who I am?"

Janet says nothing.

He prods. "C'mon, Mom, which of your sons am I? You can do it." As he speaks, Tim reminds me of a high school soccer coach giving a pep talk.

I understand he intends to be helpful and is trying to encourage his mother to remember, but this tactic is backfiring. Janet appears distraught as well as confused.

I lead them to the spacious living room where they can sit, visit and, I hope, feel more relaxed.

Janet's response to her son's questioning made me realize our role—as a relative, care partner, friend, visitor, resident assistant or other team member—includes smoothing the way for people living with dementia. We must ask ourselves how we can make life easier for them. This doesn't mean we should do things for individuals living with dementia that they can do themselves. Rather, we should not expect their brains to accomplish tasks they cannot manage, such as understanding logic, remembering previous conversations, or... recalling our names. This task will prove even more difficult if we have been absent for a while.

When we see someone using crutches due to a broken leg, are we upset that they're not meeting our expectation of walking without them? No, we have compassion for those who need help getting around, and we are happy to hold a door open to make things easier for them. Why not extend the same consideration to individuals whose brains are affected by dementia?

In an interview conducted by researcher Kim Eckart, University of Wisconsin anthropology professor Janelle Taylor questions the value of worrying about whether a person living with dementia still recognizes you. The more important question, Taylor points out, is "Do you recognize *them*?"[14] Meaning, I think, do you *see* them? Can you connect with, support, honor and befriend who they are *now*?

The interaction between Janet and her relatives taught me that my job included smoothing the way for family members to communicate with their loved ones. I could have met with the family first, without Janet, to learn how long it had been since they last saw her. I might have mentioned she may not remember their names. It would have been wise to point out that avoiding memory-related questions could ease her anxiety. Instead, they could use statements to provide helpful answers. If her son had said, "Mom, it's me, your favorite son, Tim!" it would have spared Janet the stress of a guessing game.

A fascinating insight from dementia specialist Megan Carnarius is that an individual living with Alzheimer's who appears to have forgotten their loved ones may actually still remember them. Carnarius points out that the damage in their brains can prevent them from controlling their facial expressions and showing emotion in the socially expected way.[15] For family members and friends of people living with dementia, this insight offers encouragement to keep visiting, connecting and supporting them as dementia progresses.

---

14 Kim Eckart, "Q&A: Janelle Taylor on 'Exemplary Friends' of People with Dementia," *UW News*, July 3, 2017, emeraldlakebooks.com/janelletaylor.

15 Megan Carnarius, "Companions on the Journey," presentation at Contemplative Caregiver Retreat, Natural Dharma Fellowship, Wonderwell Mountain Refuge, Springfield, New Hampshire, November 13, 2022.

Transitioning from the role of daughter, son, husband, wife, significant other, brother and so on to that of a care partner for a family member may not be easy. If you have experienced physical or emotional abuse from a parent who is now in need of care, I'd understand why you would balk at taking on the demands of the care partner role. On the other hand, I have heard moving stories of adult children who, in time, developed a loving, trusting relationship with someone who had been abusive to them earlier in life. As the parent's dementia progressed, they became more easygoing, open and affectionate. Author Deborah Cohan explores issues related to family caregiving and redemption in her memoir called *Welcome to Wherever We Are.*[16]

Asking for help with caregiving and seeking resources as needed are signs of strength, not weakness. As a family member, building a trusting relationship is essential when assuming the role of care partner. However, if this proves challenging or impossible, there is no shame in requesting advice and information from the Alzheimer's Association, a social worker, or another counselor who can guide you toward a fruitful rapport. Or you might look for resources to help you find a caregiver who can both manage your relative's care and foster a supportive, positive bond with them.

Human beings cannot thrive without meaningful relationships.

Human beings cannot thrive without meaningful relationships. I felt sad when individuals in our memory care community didn't receive regular attention from family members. Sometimes, this was due to people living far away, dealing with health issues, managing demanding jobs, and other understandable reasons. However, I wondered if certain

16 Deborah Cohan, *Welcome to Wherever We Are* (New Brunswick, NJ: Rutgers University Press, 2020).

families assumed a meaningful relationship was impossible because of the changes and challenges posed by dementia.

Memory care communities, family members, and religious groups or other neighborhood organizations can help combat the isolation and stigma that often accompany a dementia diagnosis. Care partner support groups and memory cafés—regular social gatherings for those living with dementia and their care partners—offer opportunities and resources for education, friendships and community building, all of which enhance the experiences of everyone involved.

Building trust with individuals is an essential element of person-centered care, a practice that has been championed in memory care for decades thanks to the pioneering work of Dr. Thomas Kitwood in the 1980s and '90s. This approach is based on understanding the individual's needs and preferences, respecting and valuing them, and building supportive relationships.

Kitwood envisioned the five great needs of a person living with dementia (comfort, identity, occupation, inclusion and attachment) as a flower with five petals, with the word *love* in the center as the connecting common denominator.[17]

I myself have witnessed these needs in the people living with dementia that I have known. Each individual has taught me something about one or more of Kitwood's five great needs, including how intense the need for attachment can be.

---

17 Thomas Kitwood, "The Experience of Dementia," *Aging and Mental Health 1*(1), 13–22, 1997.

Understanding Attachment

Hold thy desperate hand.
—William Shakespeare, *Romeo and Juliet*, act 3, sc. 3

Mollie

Mollie distinguished herself in our assisted living residence with her red hair, freckles and infectious laugh. She moved in soon after her husband passed away. Although she ached from missing him, her vibrant personality kept her resilient. She enjoyed talking about the countless cookies, muffins and cakes she used to bake and deliver to her family and friends. Most of all, she loved reminiscing about her weekends. For many years, every Friday and Saturday evening, she and her husband danced the night away in community ballrooms.

After about a year, Mollie's declining cognition resulted in a transfer to our memory care community. I remember when Mollie and a gentleman from assisted living danced together at a large party in the main dining room. They left their walkers behind before joining hands on the dance floor. Those of us on the care team held our breath and crossed our fingers that neither would fall. Both maintained their balance without issue as long-term memory and the joy of movement and music kicked in. Imagine the dramatic difference it made for these two to dance without nervous team members interrupting their fun, and how little the fact of living with dementia mattered to Mollie while she was dancing.

Everyone on a care team must recognize the significance of attachment for people experiencing dementia. Offering them a hand or a hug—or expressing that you could use a hug and asking if they have one to share—can help satisfy a person's need for connection, comfort and belonging. Gentle, appropriate touch is a fundamental element in fostering trusting relationships.

Mollie has developed a new habit. She squeezes her right thumb with extreme force, using the other four fingers. Her fingernails dig so far into her flesh that the skin is breaking. She keeps this pressure on for hours on end.

Mollie's daughter and our memory care nurse fail in repeated attempts to persuade her to loosen her grip. It's my turn to try.

"Mollie, do you think you could let go of that thumb just for one minute?"

"No. It's the only thing I've got." Mollie is adamant.

Her need to feel connected makes me think about all the dancing she and her husband enjoyed together. How it must hurt to miss those nights of holding onto him as they twirled around the dance floor.

While grabbing her thumb with brutal force was an unconventional way for Mollie to create a purposeful focus and maintain a sense of strength in her solitude, I appreciated her resourcefulness. She deepened my understanding that the impulse to attach oneself to others and hold tight to what gives life meaning is a significant human need—one that continues to seek expression even when a person is living with dementia.

> The impulse to attach oneself to others and hold tight to what gives life meaning is a significant human need.

I have worked with people who communicate their desire for attachment by clinging to a stuffed animal or a baby doll. I've seen others carry around a cherished photograph of their mother, a golf trophy, or another precious memento. Often, these individuals show their treasures to anyone they encounter.

A person's longing for connection is only satisfied when they have strong relationships they can count on. These are essential when navigating an individual's challenging emotions.

Responding to Intense Emotions

His passions, like a whale on ground,
Confound themselves with working.
—William Shakespeare, *II Henry IV*, act 4, sc. 4

Ida

A strong, stout, determined woman of Norwegian descent, Ida was one of my primary educators on the topic of dealing with intense emotions. Despite a rough early life and emotional fragility exacerbated by dementia, she almost reached the impressive age of 102. When Ida was eleven, her mother and younger brother died in a flu epidemic. She grew up fast, assuming the caretaker role in her motherless household and preparing all the meals.

I worked with Ida for more than ten years. On any given day, her personality could swing from frightened child to jaded wise woman to raucous comedienne. She had a robust laugh and a mischievous twinkle in her blue eyes when enjoying herself. Ida also held passionate beliefs and opinions. When collecting input to include in my thesis about the Friends InDeed project, I invited her to share her thoughts on the importance of friendship. She pondered this for a moment.

"It's so nice to have a friend stop by," she mused. With increasing fervor, she continued, "Friends are so important. We need them." All of a sudden, Ida was on the verge of tears. Making a fist, she pounded on the arm of her chair and proclaimed at the top of her voice, "We need them!"

I'm impressed by Ida's industriousness. She has figured out how to maneuver out of her apartment while sitting in her wheelchair. Since her footrests are seldom in place, she uses her feet, coupled with fierce determination, to propel herself down the hallway. Her destination is the small resident assistant office, where she hopes to find company.

If she sees no one there, she calls out in a plaintive, childlike voice, "I'm afraid." If there is no reply, she repeats, "I'm afraid. I'm afraid." She raises her voice, repeating her lament again and again, as her agitation and desperation build to "I'm crying!" (And that is not an exaggeration.)

One day, as I enter the hallway, I overhear Ida's anxiety ramping up. A couple of team members rush out of nearby apartments and go to her side. They attempt to soothe her.

"Ida, don't be afraid."

"Why are you afraid, Ida? There's nothing to be afraid of."

While these young women care for Ida and have good intentions, I realize their responses are ineffective. Instead of validating her feelings, the words they use in their attempt to calm her imply she has no reason to feel what she feels. This offers no comfort. I resolve to be the first at Ida's side next time to try a different approach.

I don't have to wait long. The following afternoon, when I enter that same hallway, Ida is calling out as before: "I'm afraid. I'm afraid."

Ida repeats this as I draw near, kneel to her eye level, and offer my hand.

"Well, Ida, of course you're afraid. You were the only person in this long, lonely hallway. But I'm here now. I'll be with you."

Ida relaxes and is happy to come along to the next activity.

A few days later, Ida is calling out in the hallway again. So I race over to her.

"I'm afraid… I'm afraid… I'm *crying*!"

Kneeling by her side, I reply, "Oh my goodness, Ida, you *are* crying. I can see the tears on your face. You must feel so sad. Tell me, what's the saddest thing for you right now?"

"I miss my dad."

"Well, of course, you miss your dad. You love him so much."

Ida's voice grows stronger. "Yes, I do. He's tops."

"Isn't he a painter?"

"Yes, he is. And a decorator too."

"A decorator too! Ida, did your dad paint every single room in your house?"

Ida is eager to tell me more. "Well, some he painted, and some he wallpapered."

"Oh, sounds like your dad has lots of skills. What color is your kitchen, Ida?

"My kitchen is yellow."

"Ooh, I like yellow for kitchens. What color is your bedroom?"

"My bedroom is pink. And it's wallpapered."

Our pleasant conversation continues for a few more minutes as Ida, eyes sparkling, shares more about her dad and his work, naming the colors he used in different rooms of their home. No trace of agitation remains in her voice, now warm and full of pride.

For a long time in dementia care, the term "redirection" (meaning diverting a person's attention to something else) was the go-to choice when people living with dementia presented challenges their caregivers preferred to avoid (such as expressing powerful emotions, wandering away from home, wondering where their deceased life partner is, thinking they have to feed the kids, wanting to search for their car, or needing to get to work). The list of such challenges is extensive because we may not always remember to devote attention and energy to *prevent* an individual's anxiety from escalating to agitation, desperation and even aggression.

When we express our understanding using some of the exact language the individual has used, hearing familiar words helps validate their point of view.

Often, we are unsure how to interact with a person living with dementia who expresses a concept of reality vastly different from ours. Early in my dementia care education, I was fortunate to hear neuropsychologist Dr. Glenn Smith, who was then with the Mayo Clinic, speak about redirection for ninety minutes at a conference. Smith explained it is a two-step process. Unless we first *join* the person and validate their perspective by acknowledging and empathizing with their feelings, whatever they may be, we have little chance of a successful redirection.[18]

18 Glenn Smith, "Validation and Redirection," presentation at the Minnesota Health and Housing Alliance, RiverCentre, Saint Paul, Minnesota, n.d.

Dementia care owes a significant debt to the late social worker and gerontologist Naomi Feil, founder of the validation approach, a method for communicating with individuals living with dementia. In a wonderful TED Talk, Feil describes this approach as "crossing to their side of the street."[19] This useful metaphor inspires me to think about how, after we make that crossing, we need to look around, see what's there, and then share our observations with the person. When we express our understanding using some of the exact language the individual has used, hearing familiar words helps validate their point of view. Efforts to redirect fail when a caregiver skips this step.

In his presentation, Smith emphasized that redirection needs to be meaningful to the person and, in fact, *equally* meaningful to their original concern.[20] Asking "Do you want a cookie?" (when you know the person who is upset is fond of them) does little to alleviate the anxiety of "I need to see my mother" unless cookies are more important to the person than their mother, which is not a safe bet. In this instance, validation before redirection could involve saying, "Of course, you want to see your mother. You miss her. Tell me more about her." You might continue this conversation for a while, then if you happen to learn about the chocolate chip cookies the person's mother used to make, you have a convenient segue into looking for treats to share.

I am grateful to Dr. Smith for this fundamental part of my dementia education and to Naomi Feil for her inspirational work on validation. Yet, it was Ida and many others living with dementia who provided ongoing proof that Smith and Feil knew precisely what they were talking about.

19 Naomi Feil, "Validation, Communication through Empathy | Naomi Feil | TEDxAmsterdamWomen," *YouTube* video, posted by TEDx Talks, June 3, 2015, emeraldlakebooks.com/naomifeil.

20 Glenn Smith, "Validation and Redirection," presentation for Minnesota Health and Housing Alliance, River Center, Saint Paul, Minnesota, n.d.

Ida's responses when discussing her dad highlight the immense power of validation. Delving into whatever is upsetting a person living with dementia offers them the assurance that someone understands. During tough times of loss or bitter disappointment, we all depend on trustworthy friends to acknowledge our feelings and needs. In the second interaction with Ida, I realized she needed at least a piece of the father she missed so much. Asking questions about her dad allowed her to brag about him and express her admiration and love. Sharing her sense of who he was reassured her that missing him and feeling such powerful emotions was normal. Of course, this was not the same as having him there, but being encouraged to talk about him was the next best thing.

I didn't have the word "validation" in my mind when, upon graduating from college with my BA in theater, I became (like ya do) a waitress for a year. I believed I was making my job more interesting when I practiced defining the overall mood of a table of people (formal, casual, celebratory, goofy and so forth) and adjusting my personality to match theirs. To my amazement, this was not only fun, but my tips increased.

When I began to work in dementia care and was getting to know individuals in our memory care community, I was reminded of my waitressing days. Since Janet seldom spoke, I communicated with her using a minimum of words. Pam, a proud, introverted and sophisticated woman, appreciated when I "invited" her to activities, employing that word rather than asking, "Do you want to go to the activity?" (Posing yes or no questions to people living with dementia, especially if they don't yet trust you, often leads to a curt reply of "no.") Babs had performed in many community theater musicals. Upon seeing her in the hallway, I would spread my arms wide and belt out "It's *Babs*!" as if I were finishing a Broadway showstopper. Laughing with abandon, she would hug me and come along to help me gather others. She needed no details about where we were going or why.

In graduate school, I was fascinated to learn that research had been conducted with Norwegian nursing students on how they interacted with those in their care. A study by Bjørg Christiansen found that drawing on different sides of oneself increased the ability to empathize with patients.[21]

In addition to adjusting our personalities for different individuals and situations, there are other tools we can use to "cross to their side of the street" when emotions run high. We can mirror people's facial expressions and gestures, keeping in mind that mirroring must remain subtle to be successful. A gentle touch conveys empathy. Commiserating with and apologizing for the person's situation are other ways to validate their feelings.

Mastering the technique of validation shouldn't seem beyond our reach. We already do this with our closest friends and family members. We celebrate their accomplishments, grieve their losses, share their joys, and feel angry or upset when they are mistreated. Without effort, we vent alongside them about challenging work issues, dysfunctional relationships, disappointments and other frustrations.

In dementia care, we often enter unfamiliar territory. While these situations may surprise us, be inconvenient, or feel uncomfortable, each presents a unique learning opportunity. Approaching challenges with curiosity and a genuine desire to help broadens our understanding of dementia and enhances our caregiving skills.

I have encountered many intense, emotional situations during my career in dementia care. Among them, my experiences with Evelyn, Ida and Essie were the most dramatic—and instructive. Their stories, which follow, each reveal something different.

---

21 Bjørg Christiansen, "Cultivating Authentic Concern: Exploring how Norwegian Students Learn this Key Nursing Skill," *Journal of Nursing Education, 48*(8), 429–33, 2009, doi.org/10.3928/01484834-20090518-03.

Essie

> For many years, Essie played the cello in a symphony orchestra. Intelligent, physically strong, and confident, she does not like being crossed. Her temper is quick, and she acts fast when protecting herself or her territory.
>
> Essie's new habit when someone annoys her is to jab them in the arm or stomach. You can always tell when she is angry enough to lash out because her cheeks flush red in an instant, and both hands become fists, ready for action.

Essie's behavior made me think about an online training with dementia care specialist Teepa Snow, in which she interacted with an upset older gentleman—let's call him Joe—who was living with dementia. Joe ran into the room where Teepa stood and straightaway pounded hard on the window glass. Teepa moved beside him and pretended to strike the wall right next to the window, displaying similar energy to Joe's. She slowed down each blow before impact, thus avoiding any harm to herself.

"I've got this, Joe," Teepa assured him. "I've got it."[22]

Joe stopped pounding. His face showed a blank look of surprise and calm. Teepa's actions and verbal reassurance had satisfied his need.

I was intrigued by how Teepa mirrored Joe's energy level while remaining below the intensity of his emotion. Showing him she was on his side in both a literal and an emotional sense calmed his distress. She had *seen* him. He was not alone.

I wondered if mirroring back intense, angry emotions would prove effective with the people I worked with, and I had the opportunity to try this out one day when Essie was rather teed off.

22 Teepa Snow, online video training, n.d.

I bring a small group of ladies, Essie among them, to join an afternoon craft activity in the memory care dining room. Unfortunately, we arrive a tad late.

As we enter, Essie glances toward her regular seat. Uh-oh. Her chair is occupied… by Evelyn. Essie's nostrils flare with annoyance.

Just as I realize I may need to intervene to prevent a confrontation, BOOM—Essie's cheeks turn red. CLICK—Her fingers curl into tight fists, poised at her side. In a split second, before she will no doubt zip across the room toward her unsuspecting target, I clench my hands at my side and step in front of Essie, facing her.

I attempt to sound as huffy and offended as possible. "Essie! I can't stand what's going on right now. Let's get out of here!" I turn and stomp out of the room, hoping she will follow. I resist looking back until I'm well into the hallway. Phew! She is just behind me.

Together, we clomp away, grumbling and sharing our mutual mood of displeasure. We rush up a flight of stairs, which poses no problem for Essie. Our pace slows down in the corridor that leads to her apartment. Once inside, we settle in for a relaxed conversation about her time with the orchestra. Before leaving, I ensure some calming classical music is playing for her to listen to.

I did not know whether that strategy would work with Essie or if I was setting myself up for a firm thump in the stomach. Yes, folks in the memory care dining room looked at me funny when I took her side and walked away in a huff with her. My colleague in charge of the craft activity was also somewhat perplexed.

Happily, no one held this aberration in my behavior against me. Once again, trying a new approach paid off.

Essie's response reaffirmed that reflecting a person's emotions can reassure them that they have an ally in a difficult moment. It's crucial to remember not to overdo the mirroring when feelings run high. With Essie, I ensured my tone of voice was energetic yet stayed below the level of her rage. Instead, I aimed to sound offended enough that she would have no reason to doubt I supported her.

Feeling isolated from friends, family and the lives they once knew can be devastating for elders living with dementia. When we show them we're on their side, they are no longer alone in whatever emotion they are experiencing, which offers considerable comfort.

Ida (Again)

Late one afternoon, Ida hovers near the secure door to the lobby in her wheelchair, distraught and pleading with me.

"I need to go. I need to catch the bus to 3634 38th Street in Minneapolis. I need to get home to make dinner for my dad!"

Until now, I have not encountered a request like this one. At a loss, I mumble about the uncertainty of the bus at this hour, which backfires, escalating Ida's distress. I need to find a way to validate her and ease her anxiety. Unsure how to accomplish this, I know I can't determine what to do with her right beside me, growing more agitated with every breath.

"Ida, wait here. I will figure this out. Give me a minute, I'll be right back."

I manage to scoot out of the memory care door into the lobby without Ida following me. I pace around, feeling pressured to find a solution before her emotions escalate further. As I near the reception desk, an idea occurs to me. I ask the receptionist for a piece of paper and a marker, then write a note as if it were a message from Ida's dad. I make the letters large and clear enough for her to read.

Uncertain how this might play out, I return to memory care. Ida, moaning and stressed, her shoulders tensed up to her ears, is waiting right where I left her.

"Ida, there was a message for you at the front desk." I read aloud from the note, which says:

> Ida, your dad called. He says to tell you that the neighbors are bringing over pot roast, mashed potatoes, and apple pie tonight. No need for you to worry about dinner.

I place the paper in Ida's hands. She looks it over. Her shoulders drop as she releases an enormous sigh. I let one out too, relieved she didn't insist on getting home for a piece of that apple pie.

Ida remains silent, seeming relaxed and comfortable as I wheel her into the dining room.

What mattered most to Ida was ensuring her dad's dinner was handled. Her response to the note confirmed that crossing to her side of the street and responding in a way that did not argue with her perception of reality was worth the gamble.

Many people feel uncomfortable lying to an individual living with dementia. I respect that. Our moral compass reminds us that telling a lie is unacceptable, particularly to those we care about. Vicki de Klerk-Rubin asserts her mother, Naomi Feil, considered this practice, known as "therapeutic fibbing," a distortion of her validation techniques.[23] Another dementia specialist, Carol Bowlby Sifton, agrees that therapeutic fibs are not ideal. She

23 Vicki de Klerk-Rubin, *Validation Techniques for Dementia Care* (Baltimore, MD: Health Professions Press, Inc., 2008), 93–4.

maintains that engaging with an individual's emotional need in the moment is a much better strategy. She also suggests that when a person is trying to find a departed loved one, reminding them they are loved and cared for is helpful.[24]

In the situation I described above, therapeutic fibbing proved effective with Ida. While I was not confident my outside-the-box idea would succeed, I had nothing to lose given Ida's level of agitation. I now find it hard to imagine what else could have alleviated her anxiety. That said, the longer I have been involved in dementia care, the less I feel the need to use therapeutic fibs. Instead, we can recognize and validate whatever emotion is true for the person before us. Our responses must align with how the person living with dementia perceives and responds to their world. If a certain task proves to be difficult for someone to accomplish, you might say, "Gosh, that's frustrating!" to acknowledge that feeling before offering help (or an easier activity). When people in my care said, "I need to see my mother" (a common complaint), I remember saying, "Of course, you miss your mother! I miss mine too." Commiserating is a handy way to validate an individual's feelings, especially when you mean it.

Honesty in dementia care has its drawbacks. Informing someone who is searching for their long-deceased partner, father or mother that their loved one has been dead for years—especially if they ask about them multiple times a day—would be cruel. Recognizing a person's emotions and providing answers that align with their current worldview is a more compassionate approach.

In the first several weeks following her husband's death, Ida would ask everyone, "Where's Roy?"

Unsure how to respond, I consulted Marie, one of our staff chaplains, who spent hours comforting Ida in her bereavement.

---

24 Carol Bowlby Sifton, *Navigating the Alzheimer's Journey* (Baltimore, MD: Health Professions Press, Inc., 2024), 98.

Marie shared what she had often told Ida in reply to that question: "Oh, Ida, I remember how Roy was so sick, and how you cared for him was wonderful. You were right there by his side the whole time."

At that point, the light would dawn, and Ida would say, "Oh, yes... And he died, didn't he?"

"Yes, that was so sad. We miss him," Marie would reply.

That script became useless, however, once Ida reached the point where she could no longer access any memory of Roy's death.

I encounter Ida in the hallway. Roy passed away several years ago, and lately, she has been asking about him every day. Right now, she is anxious and whiny. I'm concerned this may escalate.

"Where's Roy?" she demands, her voice laced with worry.

I check my watch. "Well, it's just 5 p.m. Do you think he might still be at work?"

"Maybe... Sometimes he goes to the bar after work." Ida crosses her arms and raises her eyebrows in disapproval, yet I detect a faint hint of a smile after she mentions the bar.

"Does he ever go bowling after work?"

"Well, yes, sometimes," Ida replies while pouting.

"My dad used to bowl on Thursday nights," I offer.

"Humph," retorts Ida, unimpressed.

Realizing this conversation shouldn't center on me, I take a firmer grasp of the discussion.

"You know what, Ida? Your birthday's coming up. Do you think maybe Roy could be out buying you a present?"

Ida brightens up with a big smile. "Oh, he never knows what to get me!" We share a laugh. It seems her worry about Roy has dissipated.

I roll Ida toward the dining room and ask what she hopes to have for dinner.

During the above conversation, Ida's responses confirmed that asking for *her* thoughts on Roy's whereabouts was a helpful tactic. My questions validated her perception of reality well enough to shift the mood and create space to change the subject.

Validation—Different Approaches to Try

There are various ways to validate a person's emotions. Mix and match these suggestions as appropriate:

- Say "Tell me more about that."[25]
- Repeat back what you understand to be true for the person.
- Use a few of the same words they are using.
- Start with the word "you." For example, "You seem upset."
- Start with the word "yes." For example, "Yes, how frustrating!"
- Say "Of course, you're ________" (fill in whatever emotion is being expressed).
- Translate the look on the person's face into a feeling. For example, "You seem worried."

Evelyn

It's been a long day. I need to clock out, but I'm with Evelyn in her apartment. She is in a state of agitation, approaching panic. She wants to get home to make sure her mother is

25 Snow and PAC, presentation at the Minnesota History Center.

all right and has enough to eat. I sit next to Evelyn on her bed. She stands up and paces with her walker—a neat trick, because her one-room apartment is so small she is forced to turn around often, which adds to her frustration.

I praise Evelyn for being such a caring daughter and try to reassure her that her mother is fine. I tell her that Sally, her daughter, is taking care of her grandmother's needs. Nothing I say helps Evelyn escape the grip of her extreme worry.

Finally, a validation technique that I have never used but had heard mentioned once pops into my head. I decide to try it out. As Evelyn's emotions rise, I stand and move closer to her. Before speaking, I concentrate on almost matching—but not exceeding—her energy level.

"Oh, Evelyn, I wish I had a magic wand so I could use it"—with vigor, I wave an imaginary wand back and forth—"and your mother would be here right now, and you could throw your arms around her!"

Evelyn throws her arms around me. "Oh, you're so darling!" She takes a quick inhale as I return her hug. "When this is all over, we'll still be friends, won't we?"

"Yes, Evelyn, of course. We will still be friends."

We release each other and sit back down. Evelyn is no longer focused on her mother. After a few minutes of relaxed conversation about her hometown, I give her another hug on my way out, grateful to have learned this approach worked with her.

Evelyn's response convinced me that expressing empathy and understanding by wishing aloud that things were different is a powerful validation strategy for acknowledging a person's feelings. Whether our brains are fully functioning or affected by dementia, we all need people we can rely on when times get tough—ones who will wish right alongside us that current circumstances were as we would prefer them to be.

As a family member, you may feel lost and despondent if your loved one is furious with you for taking them from their home and moving them into the unfamiliar environment of a memory care community. A loved one may complain about being isolated and out of place because everyone else is "so old" or "too crazy." Parent-child role reversal can feel awkward and unfair to both parties. Pairing a heartfelt apology with a sincere wish can be helpful in this situation: "I'm so sorry, Mom. I wish things were different." Full stop. Let that sink in. No need for an explanation or logical argument packed with bullet points about why "this is the best place for you, Mom."

The Einstein Healthcare Network explains that a "blameless apology" is one that acknowledges conditions are difficult and uncomfortable for a person. This type of apology conveys empathy and recognizes that an individual is dealing with an extreme challenge, one that is difficult for them to cope with.[26] We often use blameless apologies with friends or family during times of hardship or tragedy. "I'm so sorry for your loss," we say, aware that we were not at fault. When we extend the same compassion to persons living with dementia, apologies can go a long way to clearing the air, leaving breathing space to change the subject. "I am so sorry. That should not have happened" is another example of a blameless apology that can make an appreciable difference for someone living with dementia.

---

26 Einstein Healthcare Network, "Blameless Apologies," *Vimeo*, May 5, 2015, emeraldlakebooks.com/blamelessapology.

Forms of Comfort

Cheer thy spirit with this comfort
—William Shakespeare, *I Henry VI*, act 1, sc. 4

Validation can provide comfort when extreme or difficult emotions, such as sadness, anger, frustration or grief, are swirling. However, an emotion is not always the underlying cause of an upset. A person's distress may stem from something as simple as their surroundings—being too cold or too hot, too dark or too bright, or overwhelmed by clutter or noise. It may also arise from physical causes such as pain, hunger, dehydration or illness. At other times, the source is psychological: a yearning for connection, a desire to feel included, or a sense of disconnection from one's identity. Upsets can also result from sheer boredom due to a lack of meaningful activity. Identifying an individual's specific need in the moment is a helpful first step in determining what might bring them solace.

Comfort comes in myriad forms: a listening ear, a warm sweater, a handwritten letter in the mail (if you remember those), a shared memory, hot soup on a cold day, a poem, a song sung over the phone, a piece of chocolate. There are countless possibilities. We all have favorite things that may comfort *us*, but these remedies may leave others scratching their heads. My husband used to soothe my furrowed brow when I was stressed by grazing his fingers through my bangs and over my scalp several times. Now that he's gone, I find consolation doing this for myself as needed.

When we offer comfort in ways that are tailored to individuals living with dementia, we create a meaningful impact. Such acts tug at one's heartstrings, evoking sweet memories. The individual in need feels a grounding sensation that reminds them of their identity and preferences. A hand to hold may do the trick for someone who is not experiencing enough physical touch. When you are caring for multiple individuals, having a variety of comfort strategies in your toolbox will help determine what works best for each person.

If you have a close friend or relative living in a memory care community or skilled care center, the care team needs to know the specific strategies or personal belongings that will comfort your loved one. On the other hand, if you're a care professional, you must remember to consult family members about this upon move-in and encourage them to provide details. When an individual's care plan includes this information, making it accessible to all involved, the person has a better chance of receiving necessary comfort, resulting in an easier day for everyone.

Dementia specialist and author Jolene Brackey suggests asking a person's adult children, if available, how their parent used to comfort *them.* Their answers may provide valuable clues about what might be meaningful to the person living with dementia.[27] Brackey also recommends having family members create and

27 Jolene Brackey, presentation at the Ebenezer Corporate Office, Edina, Minnesota, April 2, 2020.

bring in a memory box, a collection of familiar items that have meaning for their loved one. These objects promote comfort, stimulate reminiscing, and encourage engagement.[28]

Reflecting on what you would like to include in your own memory box is an enjoyable exercise. One day when my sinuses were congested, I remembered I had some Vicks VapoRub in the closet. (Ancient VapoRub. Good grief! The expiration date was fifteen years earlier!) I was amazed that the little jar still released an intense aroma, providing my nose, chest and throat with that familiar, tingly cool, mentholated sensation. The scent transported me back to my childhood bedroom, gazing at the blue and white patterned wallpaper on the gabled walls. I recalled times when I was sick and Mom would serve me milk toast in bed, which sounds terrible now but was soothing and delicious then. What would you include in your memory box?

Whether you work in assisted living, memory care, or adult daycare, or are caring for someone at home, your comfort needs should not be ignored. Practicing self-care is an essential support for yourself and will benefit those you care for. It can be tough, however, to take enough breaks for rest, relaxation and physical and mental well-being. You need to be willing to ask for help when necessary.

If you're caring for someone at home and a friend says, "Let me know if you need anything," before they hurry off, why not pull out a prepared list of ways they could assist you? Be specific. For instance, "Come play checkers with my husband next Tuesday from two to four p.m.," or "I'm all out of dark chocolate."

28 Jolene Brackey, *Creating Moments of Joy Along the Alzheimer's Journey*, 5th ed. (West Lafayette, IN: Purdue University Press, 2017), 184–85.

Ida

Sometimes, a person living with dementia will experience a sudden upset at an inopportune time for you, their caregiver. If an individual is away from their familiar environment, this can escalate their distress. In such situations, you may need to improvise to find a solution that provides effective relief and comfort.

Ida whimpers as I wheel her out of the main dining room and onto the elevator, leaving our monthly birthday party behind. Today, she can't tolerate the cacophony and commotion. Many members of our memory care community attend, and she has always held up well, until now.

Ida's anxiety increases as we descend to the lobby. I rack my brain for words to say or what to do to help her calm down. She is on the verge of tears when the elevator doors slide open.

I plead with a team member crossing our path to stay with Ida in the lobby for a minute while I try to find something that might help. She agrees.

Walking as fast as possible without running, I pass through the memory care doors and dash down the hall to the activity room to grab what I need. Soon, a cloth doll with floppy arms and legs, yellow braids and a happy face accompanies me as I stride back to the lobby. It is about the size of a seven-year-old child and was donated a week ago. I've wondered whether it would appeal to anyone in our memory care community.

I rush into the lobby, where Ida's distress level has escalated several notches. "Ida, look what I found," I announce, placing the enormous smiling doll on her lap.

"Aww!" In an instant, Ida's demeanor transforms. She hugs the doll close with a sweet smile. I only have time for a relieved exhale before Ida commands, "Take a picture."

We have a camera at the reception desk, making it easy to obey Ida's directive. I capture her and her new friend in a cheerful mood of complete calm.

I did not know whether a gigantic cloth doll could make a significant change in Ida's mood. For all I knew, she might have thrown it back at me and started to scream.

The better you understand the people in your care and the more you learn about what brings them happiness and comfort, the more accurate your instincts become in making a dramatic difference for them.

The better you understand the people in your care and the more you learn about what brings them happiness and comfort, the more accurate your instincts become in making a dramatic difference for them.

Mom

As I mentioned earlier, Mom adored babies. For many years, her purpose in life was to run a household, care for her husband, raise five children, and dote on her grandchildren and great-grandchildren.

These days, memory care sites often offer a collection of life-like baby dolls for individuals living with dementia to admire, cradle, rock, carry around, talk to and find comfort in. One of our Ebenezer communities dedicates an entire room to The Nursery, which includes several bassinets, rocking chairs, and numerous baby dolls. I've observed women there caring for their "babies" and bringing them to activities. While some women find simple comfort from holding and admiring the dolls, others seem transported back in time, feeling younger than their actual age and reliving their purpose.

When I started in dementia care, I wanted to give Mom a baby doll. I learned they were common in these environments, and I hoped a doll might provide soothing engagement for her. However, my brother and sister were adamant this was beneath Mom's dignity. Despite my recent plunge into dementia care, as the youngest sibling, living far away, and not one of Mom's family contacts, my chances of winning that argument were nil. So, I did not pursue it.

Many years later, when Mom was at her final residence, a nursing home, she received extra engagement and attention from a private caregiver named Marcy, a woman who was animated, chatty and savvy. When she discovered Mom's love for babies, she decorated my mother's bathroom door with pictures of infants of various ages, skin colors and sizes, each displaying a different facial expression. These images were sizable; Marcy cut them from magazines or found them on large greeting cards. Mom could see them well from her bed. She must have spent hours communing with those faces.

I arrive at the nursing home after flying in from Minnesota. When I walk into Mom's room, she is engrossed in the gallery of baby faces on the bathroom door and doesn't notice me. I sit and watch as she murmurs to each one in turn, taking time to mimic their facial expressions. (I realize she is validating their feelings!)

After about fifteen minutes, I capture Mom's attention. She lets me apply lotion to her hands, but she isn't as interested in me or my hand massage as she was in the baby faces. I'm glad she has these pictures to keep her company.

Sometimes, a familiar memory will comfort an individual. When Mom was more verbal, she enjoyed telling a funny story about my brother, Bob. His regular chore was to take out the garbage. Our driveway sloped down to the garage at the back of our house, near the trash cans. Bob liked to set up an open can at the bottom of the driveway and launch the large garbage bag from the landing outside our kitchen. He became skilled at always making a basket with the trash, but one time, when Mom, Dad and I all happened to be watching, he missed. The bag split open, scattering its contents across the driveway. Mom became helpless with laughter when she described how she and Dad were cracking up while Bob slunk off to clean up the mess.

Over time, Mom stopped being the one to offer this story. If I asked her about that time with Bob and the garbage in the driveway, she would share it and laugh. As she became less verbal, I began to tell it, then she would chime in and take over right before the bag split open. At a certain point, I told her the story from start to finish. She listened with interest and smiled at the end every time.

My mother's fondness for recalling this event showed me that as dementia progresses, it's important to help those in our care revisit cherished, humorous and meaningful memories that bring comfort and smiles.

Ollie

Of course, it wasn't Ollie's idea to move from assisted living to memory care. Such discussions can be challenging for families, but his sons were both kind and candid when they spoke with him about his cognitive changes. Ollie, a calm and intelligent gentleman, agreed receiving extra help at this time was a wise decision.

> On moving day, I'm impressed by how Ollie's family engages him in the physical move. They are transferring his belongings together, making multiple trips back and forth from his assisted living apartment on the third floor to his new place

on the first. Each time, his walker is loaded with books and smaller items.

Ollie's acceptance of his situation and cheerful participation in the move contributed to the smoothest transition from assisted living to memory care I have ever witnessed. He showed that, like the rest of us, people living with dementia want and need to feel useful. The simple act of being helpful can be a source of comfort.

During a transition to memory care, the assisted living team members who collaborate with families to support those with dementia have the right idea. Not everyone will be as enthusiastic and able as Ollie, but even those confined to a wheelchair could perhaps help by holding a few items on their laps. With forethought and creativity, people's strengths and skills can be acknowledged and utilized on moving day.

Once settled into his new, smaller space, Ollie was content to stay occupied with the books and papers on his handsome wooden desk, where, as an accountant, he had crunched many numbers. While he participated in occasional music activities, he tended to keep to himself when he wasn't receiving attention from his devoted sons.

Ollie has a new routine. Each morning after breakfast, he sits on his bed for thirty to forty-five minutes. He leaves his apartment door wide open in case anyone wants to listen to him sing the Irish ballads he learned at his mother's knee. These are obscure tunes, not ones we are used to hearing or singing on St. Patrick's Day.

I marvel how Ollie finds pleasure, relaxation and comfort in revisiting these ditties every morning. Singing these songs from his childhood is an excellent exercise for his brain, and everyone who passes through the hallway is enchanted enough to stop in their tracks to listen.

Ollie was fortunate to retain the skills and resourcefulness he needed to engage himself in meaningful ways. Imagine being unable to initiate activities related to your current interests and passions. If I could no longer pick up a pen, use a computer, or organize my thoughts, the prospect of writing a book would feel mighty discouraging. Without the ability to get myself to the theater now and then, I would be miserable. And if I could no longer hop on an airplane to visit family or distant friends, my world would feel small and sad. However, with support, I might still work on a book project, attend the theater, and figure out ways to travel.

Creating Engaging Activities

We have had pastimes here and pleasant game.
—William Shakespeare, *Love's Labour's Lost*, act 5, sc. 2

Linda

People who live with dementia have a rich history of experiences and accomplishments. This wealth of skills and memories must be accessed, stimulated and transformed into successful engagement opportunities. Understanding which pursuits have been most significant to an individual throughout their life is an excellent step to develop activities that will bring them joy.

As dementia progresses, people tend to slow down and often become less verbal. If a person cannot recall your name or is not as animated as they once were, you might suppose with a sigh that they aren't "there" anymore and conclude they have forever lost interest in things that once occupied their attention and brought them happiness. This is a dangerous assumption. The heart remains intact, remember? A passion for a former activity may diminish due to uncertainty about how or where to begin, or from the pain of being unable to perform as well as one used to.

Linda's profound sorrow regarding the cognitive changes she faces is evident. A newcomer to our memory care community and younger than most who live here, she often visits my office early in the morning to chat. Petite, with clear blue eyes and short, wavy silver hair, Linda dresses in artsy, stylish clothing. She shares stories about her painting career and yearns for the art studio in her previous home.

Eager to give Linda an outlet for her talent, I hire a local artist experienced in leading creative activities for elders to run a series of painting sessions for memory care folks in our activity room.

Linda is excited to attend the first session, but it fast becomes clear that the project is too simple to hold her interest. Moreover, it's painful for her to realize her mind, instincts and paintbrush no longer collaborate as they used to. Frustrated and discouraged, she declines invitations to return to ongoing sessions.

Linda still had a tremendous passion for painting, but her mind struggled to navigate the obstacle course that dementia had erected in her brain. Our art group activity must have felt to her like being sent back to kindergarten. Hindsight suggests that a private session with a more sensitive teacher might have been more valuable, and I regret not considering this option at the time.

While "loss of initiative" is listed among the symptoms of dementia, I believe "loss of interest in activities people once enjoyed" should not be included without further explanation. Let's not assume someone has lost their passion for an activity or hobby just because they feel frustrated by losing the physical or mental abilities that once gave them confidence. Linda was stymied by her inability to paint as she once did, but her face shone with excitement during an outing to an art gallery she had frequented in the past. Art remained an essential part of her identity.

I asked Linda's daughter, Jen, for insight into hobbies or pastimes beyond painting that had brought her mom happiness. Jen did not have to think before answering, and I was glad I'd asked. "Clouds. My mom was always fascinated by and drawn to clouds."

In addition, Jen revealed Linda had earned her pilot's license decades ago and enjoyed flying a small plane. No wonder clouds entranced her. I bet she painted many pictures of them during those years when she was both a pilot and a painter.

I've cut various cloud shapes out of white felt. As attendees arrive, they each take a shape to stick onto a light blue background.

After we listen to Simon and Garfunkel's song "Cloudy," I share poems about clouds. We discuss different types of formations and recall how, as children—and perhaps beyond—we enjoy spotting familiar shapes in them. Linda is attentive and appreciative.

A few weeks later, Jen is pleased to lead an activity about her mom's experience as a pilot. She brings a heavy box filled with photos and memorabilia to share with our group, including a newspaper article featuring a large picture of Linda, grinning over her shoulder in the cockpit of a plane. She smiles that way now, describing how amazing it felt to fly right up into and above the clouds.

Individuals living with dementia are often eager to engage in activities related to their interests, hobbies and cherished pursuits. Some may jump at the chance to help plan a presentation on a familiar topic; others might favor spontaneous discussion and reflection about their specific passions.

Memory care communities in Minnesota must identify the activities people have loved and the accomplishments that have brought them joy and purpose. Engagement opportunities tied to individuals' interests must be included on the events calendar, and documenting activity attendance is mandatory. While Minnesota is a trailblazer in this area, it's unfortunate all fifty states don't have such explicit laws addressing dementia care. However, I look forward to the day when many more US states commit to ensuring personalized activities are available for those living with dementia.

I have known introverts living in memory care who hesitate to join group activities. Others may resist because they are not yet accustomed to community living. People need time to adjust to new surroundings. In a memory care community, this takes between three weeks and three months, in my experience. Having individualized activities on the schedule is one way to attract those who might not otherwise attend. People might decide to come when they hear the activity features their seatmate at dinner or because a new offering sounds intriguing. I found a reliable selling point in reminding folks that learning new things is one of the best things you can do for your brain.

Family members were delighted to find their loved one's name attached to an activity on the calendar. Following the success of "My Life as a Pilot with Linda," I decided we needed to add "Pole Vaulting with Betsy" next month.

Betsy

I enjoy referring to Betsy Macfee as "The Amazing Betsy Macfee" because she was an accomplished pole vaulter during her high school and college years. Betsy, who is tall, easygoing, independent and disciplined, now uses a walker without complaint.

At my request, our receptionist finds time to print photos of famous pole vaulters from the 1940s and '50s. I collect fun facts about pole vaulting to share along with the photos.

During the activity, our on-site expert, Betsy, holds court to answer our questions.

"Betsy, how did jumping that high feel?"

"Fun."

"How high did you jump?"

"Oh, twelve or thirteen feet, maybe."

"Did you have to practice every day?"

"Oh yes, almost. I think so." Betsy's replies are not elaborate, but her eyes twinkle as she responds to our queries. It's clear she is proud to share this part of herself.

Betsy was remarkable in other ways too. She was the one person in our community with no interest in drinking coffee. Green tea was gaining recognition for its health benefits, and she requested it at every meal.

Her husband, an attorney whom she described as "a very kind man," passed away when she was in her early fifties. To cope with her loss, she had picked herself up and traveled the world all on her own.

Sometimes, in an impromptu group, we play "Let's Stump Betsy." In turn, everyone in our circle names a different country, and she tells us whether she has traveled there. Her answers are impressive.

She either says, "Yes, I've been there" or "Yup, I think so."

Caring for individuals living with dementia involves a significant responsibility to provide meaningful opportunities for activity. Linda and Betsy taught me that the things we cherish most in our lives give tremendous pride and satisfaction. When we explore these interests and achievements with those in our care, we engage with them on a deeper level.

> The things we cherish most in our lives give tremendous pride and satisfaction.

Ida

Proud of her Norwegian heritage, Ida was thrilled when I planned a party to celebrate the anniversary of Syttende Mai. This holiday commemorates May 17, 1814, when King Christian VIII (then Prince Christian Frederik) signed the Norwegian constitution, leading to Norway's independence from Denmark.

I asked Ida what food we should serve at this party. She knew right away what to suggest: traditional Serinakaker butter cookies.

"Okay," I gulped, hoping I could find out how to spell that… and find a bakery that makes them.

Visiting a Scandinavian bakery the day before the party, I learn they don't carry those cookies. I find a recipe online and bake two dozen. When I take them out of the oven, they look a bit heavy. I cross my fingers—maybe they are meant to be dense. Still, I have my doubts.

The next day, the hefty appearance of the cookies doesn't deter Ida from biting into one with gusto. As she chomps, her jaw moves slower… and slower.

"They're a little chewy."

What an understatement! Ida's comment is garbled due to the challenge in her mouth. I'm relieved when she manages to wash it down with lemonade with no ill effects.

Ida's excitement for this holiday, an integral part of her cultural identity, touches me. After sneaking the cookies away, I guide guests to other snacks.

Another day, Ida reminisces about the hardware store she and Roy owned and managed together. She tells us they had just one employee, who worked alongside them for years.

Knowing how fond Ida was of the store, I give her a thick four-inch bolt and a matching nut to fit together. Her eyes, weakened by macular degeneration, are not much help. The smaller nuts and bolts I tried with her before caused frustration. I'm hoping the bigger hardware will be easier for her to manipulate. For a full ten minutes, Ida concentrates on getting that chunky nut onto the big bolt. I watch as she feels her way to make the grooves fit together. She succeeds, releasing a satisfied breath of accomplishment.

Observing her effort, I start to grasp why, at nearly one hundred years old, Ida is still with us. She is the essence of perseverance. Having worked throughout most of her long life, she thrived on getting tasks done that needed doing. Ida and Roy dedicated themselves to their small business, which served their community well. How she loves being reminded of all this now!

In addition to creating activities based on individual experiences, interests and family heritage, it's always a good idea to focus on what will bring fun and enjoyment to those in your care.

The Joy of Cookies, Bacon and Music

O, rejoice
Beyond a common joy, and set it down
With gold on lasting pillars
—William Shakespeare, *The Tempest*, act 5, sc. 1

Gloria

When you think of dementia, joy is probably not the first word that pops into your mind. Despite the undeniable challenges cognitive decline may pose, that does not mean that a person is destined to lose the capacity to laugh and enjoy life. That "muscle" may not have been exercised for a while, so naturally, it could be out of practice. Beyond reminding those in our care of what they love and what they are fond of remembering, well-chosen activities can provide a source of exhilaration—or a sweet, simple sense of returning to something important and precious.

Gloria's enthusiastic heart radiates hope and optimism. With deep pride, she finds strength and comfort sharing stories about her large family, her strong Catholic faith, her fond memories of founding a YMCA in Yorkville, Illinois, and… her famous oatmeal cookie recipe.

Gloria's favorite story to tell features Bob Hope, the renowned comedian and dedicated entertainer of troops overseas. They met at a fundraiser for missionaries that her husband had organized. She offered Mr. Hope one of her homemade cookies, which he was pleased to accept. She was eager to hear his review.

Bob took a few bites in silence, then announced, "This is the best damn cookie I ever ate!"

When Gloria tells this story, she laughs with abandon and repeats the punchline: "Best damn cookie I ever ate!"

I bet Bob received a second cookie. Why didn't I ever ask Gloria's daughter for the recipe back then? That was a missed opportunity. Making those cookies in our baking group and hearing the story while munching on them would have been fun.

Thankfully, I was able to get Gloria's recipe from her daughter while writing this book. So, just in case there are still some Bob Hope fans out there who might appreciate these oatmeal cookies, I'm sharing the recipe with you here.

Gloria's Oatmeal Cookies

Preparation Time: 15 minutes
Baking Time: 15–16 minutes
Oven Temperature: 350°F
Yield: 2 dozen cookies

Ingredients:

1½ sticks (¾ cup) butter

2 cups sugar

2 eggs

1 tsp cinnamon

1 tsp nutmeg

1 tsp baking soda

2½ cups flour

4 tbsp milk

7½ oz raisins

2 cups oatmeal

Gloria's Tip:
Store cookies in an air-tight container with a slice of bread to keep them soft and moist for several days.

Preparation:

1. Preheat the oven to 350°F.
2. In a large bowl, mix together the butter, sugar and eggs until creamy.
3. In a second bowl, combine the cinnamon, nutmeg, baking soda and flour.
4. Slowly add the dry ingredients and milk to the butter mixture while blending.
5. Stir in the raisins and oatmeal.
6. Drop dough by spoonfuls onto a greased cookie sheet.
7. Bake for 15–16 minutes.

Notes:

- This recipe can easily be doubled.
- The dough freezes well.

Mom

> Mom doesn't speak much these days. She has been in hospice care for over a year. This morning, her primary caregiver is wheeling her down to breakfast. As they approach the dining room, all of a sudden, Mom sits up straight, sniffs a few times, and pronounces with approval, "Bacon!"

Sometime after Mom's diagnosis of "probable Alzheimer's disease," she was also diagnosed with Parkinson's disease. While Parkinson's is often associated with a reduced sense of smell, this was no obstacle for my mother that morning.

Over the years, she had crisped up plenty of bacon for her husband and five children. During my high school days, every Thursday evening, Mom and I crumbled it on our baked potatoes, along with broccoli and cheddar cheese. The two of us were on our own for dinner on Dad's bowling night since all my siblings were out of the house by then.

I wonder if the olfactory stimulation wafting down the hallway that morning, many decades later, triggered memories for Mom of being in her kitchen on Sunday mornings, with family members hovering nearby, eager for breakfast. In addition to enjoying that enticing smell, I hope she felt a warm sense in her heart for those she fed, cared for and loved.

> The more we tailor activities to resonate with a person's fondest memories, the greater the impact on their well-being.

I still take pleasure in preparing a baked potato with broccoli and cheddar cheese, and yes, sometimes bacon, because of those dinners Mom and I shared.

Sensory stimulation is an essential element of engagement for people living with dementia. My Tales from a Trunk audiences proved that the more we incorporate things they can see, hear, touch, smell or taste into our activities, the more likely they are to participate.

Working in memory care, I came to understand that the level of engagement in any activity, including personal hygiene, also depends on the quality of the human interaction surrounding it.

Activities should not be mere fillers used to pass time until the next meal; instead, they should offer opportunities to recall precious memories, stimulate and stretch the brain, and provide individuals living with dementia with a tangible sense of purpose.

The more we tailor activities to resonate with a person's fondest memories, the greater the impact on their well-being.

Fran

Fran is a cheerful, energetic woman with a ready laugh. She adores music, has a captivating singing voice, and loves sharing her talent. She knows every verse and many of the lesser-known introductions to countless songs from the 1930s, '40s and '50s. Walking down the hallway or alone in her apartment, Fran hums and sings to herself. When anything mentioned in conversation reminds her of a tune, she breaks into song. All present are happy to follow her lead.

Award-winning journalist and novelist John Colapinto reports music has been among the most successful ways to help a person hold on to memories in the face of Alzheimer's disease. His exploration of this topic recognizes music as a "full-brain workout" that lights up the brain stem, motor centers, language centers, auditory cortex, visual systems, and emotional centers. Familiar, beloved music provides people living with dementia with a sense of orientation to the present and deepens their connection to their own identity.[29]

Whether in assisted living, memory care, a nursing home, or at home, people living with dementia benefit from the use of a voice-activated assistant (like Alexa or Siri), personalized iPods with headphones, CD players, or whatever equipment they have available for entertainment. Establishing a regular time each day when caregivers ensure individuals have time to enjoy their favorite music is an excellent idea. Meaningful engagement doesn't have to happen in a group.

Ted

Ted was struggling to adjust to his new home—a modest room in a large memory care community—and was resisting personal care (bathing, dressing, grooming, etc.). A respected academic who spoke four languages, he was accustomed to a cultured life.

I was asked to meet with Ted, observe personal care, and provide suggestions to his care team. When I arrived early one morning to meet him, a colleague of mine, someone Ted trusted, introduced us. After she had to scurry away, Ted and I chatted. I wasn't surprised when he seemed uneasy with me, this stranger who had been left alone with him with little explanation.

> Ted has an Alexa smart speaker in his apartment. My colleague mentioned Ted is a devoted fan of classical music, in particular, Rachmaninoff's Concerto No. 2 in C Minor, Op. 18. Since chatting is not getting us anywhere, I ask Alexa to play it. Right on cue, majestic, sweeping, euphoric music emerges from the speaker.

29 John Colapinto, "The Extraordinary World of Music and the Mind," *AARP The Magazine*, January 2024, 49–56.

> The effect is magical. Ted relaxes, and so do I. He is more comfortable with my presence, and we have more to discuss once the music concludes.

As it turned out, there was no opportunity for me to observe Ted's personal care during my visit. However, I recommended care team members make it a habit to ask Alexa for this specific music during personal care and whenever he needs comfort or engagement.

My experiences with Ted and Fran reinforced what many others living with dementia have shown me: Music is a reliable pathway to understanding a person's heart and spirit. Dr. Stephen G. Post, Director of the Center for Medical Humanities, Compassionate Care and Bioethics and author of two groundbreaking books on dementia, asserts people living with cognitive decline benefit from having daily access, one way or another, to *their* music, music that provides them with hope, comfort, joy, relaxation and memories.[30]

Identify Their Favorite Things

Knowing what people's favorite things are helps in planning engaging activities. Having a group discussion to discover this information is a fun activity in itself. On a large whiteboard, list answers in selected categories, such as: favorite song, favorite beverage, favorite color, favorite sound, favorite ice cream flavor, favorite food, favorite smell or scent, favorite weather, favorite sport, favorite sports team, favorite holiday, favorite hobby, favorite artist, favorite singer, favorite poet, favorite

30 Stephen G. Post, "Closing Plenary and Discussion with Panelists Living with Dementia," presentation at Dementia Action Alliance Conference, Crowne Plaza Hotel, Indianapolis, Indiana, September 21, 2022.

author, favorite animal, favorite comedian, favorite flower, favorite subject in school, favorite musical, favorite place to visit, favorite season, favorite summer activity, favorite winter activity, favorite thing to do with a friend…

Engagement with Purpose

Here is the heart of my purpose
—William Shakespeare, *The Merry Wives of Windsor*, act 2, sc. 2

I well remember, many years ago, walking into my bedroom to check on my twelve-month-old daughter. Eliza had been crawling around and quiet for too long. I discovered her ripping up the pages of a stack of picture books stored on an open bottom shelf of a nightstand. Grinning from ear to ear, sitting amid a messy pile of shredded paper, she was having a blast with her newfound accomplishment.

Children are curious. Their brains are designed to pursue activities that interest them, build motor skills, and offer a sense of achievement. People living with dementia tend to lose skills in the reverse order of how children gain them as they grow. Although those who experience dementia are full-fledged adults, as the condition progresses, their brains respond to their environment as though from an earlier developmental stage. In her book, *A Deeper Perspective on Alzheimer's and Other Dementias,*

Megan Carnarius explores this progressive journey with profound insight and compassion.[31]

We need to stay aware that the minds of those living with dementia will seek ways to remain engaged and to experience the satisfaction of fulfilling a purpose. We must also remember that we may or may not appreciate the plan those minds design.

Marlene

Marlene is tall, stunning, well-read and sophisticated. Her apartment is full of furniture and fascinating artifacts from years spent living and traveling overseas with her diplomat husband. Despite her dementia, Marlene is vibrant and clever. She often turns to rhyming to liven things up or keep herself entertained.

I've gathered a group of five ladies for a spontaneous activity. I'm sharing photos from a booklet designed to stimulate reminiscences. Marlene is bored. She interrupts our discussion with rhymes for any words in our conversation that catch her attention.

Since her rhyming is impossible to ignore and reminiscing doesn't seem to be taking off for anyone, I switch gears. I compliment Marlene on her ability and say, "Marlene, I wonder if you could make up a rhyme for each of us in this group. I'll say the name, and you give me a rhyme for it, okay?"

Marlene is all in. Our conversation is about to get livelier.

31 Megan Carnarius, *A Deeper Perspective on Alzheimer's and other Dementias,* (Findhorn, Scotland: Findhorn Press, 2015).

Here's how it went:

MARYSUE: Fran.

MARLENE: Fran has a man.

(Fran couldn't be more delighted.)

MARYSUE: Gerry.

MARLENE: Gerry is very merry.

MARYSUE: Bernice.

MARLENE: Bernice fell in the grease.

MARYSUE: Meg.

MARLENE: Meg has a funny leg.

MARYSUE: Dottie.

MARLENE: (without hesitation) Dottie, Dottie, two by four, can't fit through the bathroom door!

(I can't help feeling grateful that Dottie, bless her, is utterly deaf and takes no offense.)

MARYSUE: Marysue.

MARLENE: Marysue, how do you do?

MARYSUE: Fine, thanks for asking! Marlene.

MARLENE: Marlene is queen.

(We all applaud.)

Another time, in the middle of a balloon volleyball game, as she is whacking the balloon over the net, Marlene belts out, "If you get to heaven before I do, just drill a hole and pull me through!" This gets a hearty laugh of appreciation from both teams. Inspired by this encouragement, Marlene repeats the phrase every few minutes and continues to say it several times each day.

Marlene's habit of rhyming was not a problem for anyone. Her audience often found her as amusing as she found herself.

Barbara

> A dementia-fueled hallucination doesn't indicate there is nothing of value or meaning occurring.

Barbara lived with Lewy body dementia and experienced recurring hallucinations. One hallucination specific to this type of dementia is seeing children or small animals running around a room. Another is believing there are bugs all over the walls or elsewhere.

Barbara is adamant she must "watch the kids" who are "running around in here." A quiet, independent sort, she moved in last week. Aside from going to meals, Barbara has not ventured out of her apartment. Encouraging her to take part in activities is a no-go proposition.

A devoted mother to several grown daughters, Barbara enjoys being in charge of the children she sees in her room and feels it's her responsibility to supervise them.

While I would love for her to socialize more, her sense of obligation is impossible to contradict. So, I say, "Well, Barbara, if those kids cause you any trouble, please let me know."

I'm grateful she sees children running and crawling around her space rather than bugs, although getting someone out of their apartment is much easier when they are convinced there is an infestation.

Barbara helped me understand that a dementia-fueled hallucination doesn't indicate there is nothing of value or meaning occurring. Her commitment to looking out for "the kids" gave her a sense of pride and much-needed purpose.

Mom

Many of us who have worked in memory care have encountered more than one person who packs up their belongings again and again because they feel it is time to "go home."

When Mom moved into her first memory care community, she was a regular packer-upper since she had it in her head she was about to be "thrown out." My brother had thought it best to tell Mom about the impending move a few weeks before the event, but this backfired. Her feeling of being thrown out of her home moved right along with her to her new place and stuck around for a while.

Over the years, I learned that, in this situation, helping someone pack is often the best way to "cross to their side of the street." Then, it's easy to suggest taking a break for lunch or an upcoming activity, while another team member goes in and unpacks. Away from their space, the person may well forget about packing, at least for the day.

Hal

Sometimes, people living with dementia channel their boredom, frustration or lack of engagement in far more challenging directions.

Hal is a cheerful, good-natured guy obsessed with hoarding paper products. A former tax attorney, he is polite when making his daily request for extra napkins in the dining room. He scores a few each time, as we have learned it's best to avoid an argument with this particular attorney.

He also collects toilet paper rolls from the hallway bathrooms. Some of his stash of paper goods is stored in haphazard fashion on shelves in his apartment. The rest gets stuffed into his toilet in epic proportions.

Another time, a woman in our memory care community called 911 for help because she felt trapped and lonesome to the point that she didn't know what else to do.

On several occasions, a different woman pulled the fire alarm. Looking back, I wonder if she acted out of desperation, panic, a desire for excitement, or a curiosity that compelled her to follow the instructions on the handle, which of course said "PULL." Regardless, it's clear that a lack of meaningful activity influenced her choice of engagement.

Bill

When Bill first arrived at our memory care residence, I knew little about him, but I soon learned he was handy with a screwdriver. He'd moved in with one in his possession. Our team failed to notice this until Bill decided to put that tool to good use.

> In broad daylight, unbeknownst to anyone working on the second floor, Bill disassembles and removes the mechanism that keeps the secure door locked and the alarm functioning. Once he exits into assisted living, it isn't long before he is intercepted and returned.
>
> Our maintenance staff drag over a hefty bookcase to block the doorway, ensuring Bill and other memory care community members remain safe and in place until the alarm mechanism is repaired.
>
> It's fortunate a second door escaped the wrath of Bill's screwdriver, which, alas for him, has now been confiscated.

Decades after Bill's escape attempt, I am encouraged and excited by the growing movement of senior communities in the US and beyond that have stopped locking the doors that divide memory care residences from assisted living. Instead, they are implementing new methods and technologies to ensure resident safety. In addition, more sites have ended the practice of segregating those needing memory care from those who don't by providing services for those living with dementia throughout the broader community. No doubt Bill would approve.

A Sense of Purpose

The actions I've described in this chapter that posed challenges for care team members made sense and were meaningful to those determined to carry them out. Recalling these incidents, I cannot help but exclaim, "Good God!" The driving force we humans feel to live a decent, interesting life, to have agency, to make decisions for our well-being, to follow self-protective instincts, to improve our lot using whatever skills (and tools) we possess, to feel free, to be free—these impulses are normal and powerful. Dementia does not snuff them out… Not by a long shot.

> Each summer, we bring women from our memory care community into our adult day center to join forces with others who are there to shuck corn. Hands are sanitized, aprons are donned, and newspaper pages are spread across long tables that have been pushed together.
>
> Talk about a sense of purpose! For well over an hour, we shuck enough corn to feed everyone in assisted living and memory care. Ladies who seem far too frail for the work channel a strength they have not exercised in years. Their skill snaps back into place as they work with fiery determination.
>
> During dinner, the women in memory care are pleased to be reminded that they helped prepare the corn that graces their plates.

These events convinced me that individuals living with dementia will not thrive without purposeful engagement, an essential support for maintaining a person's overall well-being, right alongside food and water.

Recognizing Meaningful Engagement

Can this be true?

—William Shakespeare, *Much Ado about Nothing*, act 3, sc. 1

Evelyn

Most Saturdays, I can convince Evelyn to come along to balloon volleyball, but all the way there, she worries aloud about her mother. Today is no different. Although she hasn't yet reached the level of panic, the storm clouds are gathering.

I do my best to reassure her, letting her know she has plenty of time to participate in the game and that we will figure everything else out later.

Evelyn keeps trudging along, repeating her litany as she pushes her walker down the hallway. "I need to get home. I need to see my mother. I need to make sure she has enough food."

Eventually, I will learn from her daughter that Evelyn had been the caregiver for her mother, who also lived with Alzheimer's disease.

Once we get to the main activity room, where people are waiting for the game to begin, I guide Evelyn to an empty front-row seat before offering to park her walker to the side.

"No charge," I tell her, which brings a smile.

Everyone is assembled. I press the play button on the boombox to start ragtime piano music by Knuckles O'Toole, who, in my opinion, provides superb accompaniment for balloon volleyball—a wonderful, bouncy soundtrack for the game.

As the balloon travels back and forth across our makeshift net, Evelyn transforms into what I can only describe as a cat watching a bird. She is competitive, focused and especially pleased with herself when she slams that balloon down over the net with a ferocity that belies her fragility. Laughing with wicked pleasure, she smiles with pride when she wins a point for the team—no one cares that we're not keeping score. She is involved in the game from start to finish.

Today, we play for a full hour. When it's time to stop, I shut off the music. We applaud our efforts, and I return people's walkers, one by one.

When I give Evelyn hers, it seems that the moment she curls her fingers around the handlebars, her anxiety creeps back in.

"Oh, I need to get home," Evelyn says. Her tone is vague and a bit surprised, but not too anxious—at least, not yet. "I need to see my mother," she continues with a tinge more worry. "I need to make sure she has enough food." She is still more relaxed, though, than when she expressed the same concerns on the way to balloon volleyball.

I'm glad she is amenable to coming to snack time, a dependable distraction after a vigorous game.

After this, a realization hits me: When people living with cognitive decline engage in experiences they enjoy, dementia doesn't hold them back in any way. During the game, Evelyn was free from her worries and the deficits related to changes in her brain. She had an entire hour in which she could simply be herself.

Hal

Hal attended the interactive, Tales from a Trunk–style activity I led one evening in late October. Halloween-themed props were passed around, costume pieces were available for those who volunteered to wear them, and we recited "Double, double toil and trouble; fire burn and cauldron bubble" from Shakespeare's spookiest play, *Macbeth*. We discussed Halloween traditions and the costumes we wore or made for our kids. I shared some corny Halloween jokes and taught the group a simple song called "Have You Seen the Ghost of Tom," which works as a round. We tried to sing it that way, but it turned into a hilarious mess since I was leading both parts.

The activity has concluded. I'm picking up scattered props and costume pieces and packing them back into my trunk. People seemed to have had fun—they applauded at the end—but now it's strange how nobody is making a move to leave. They seem unworried about where to go or what will happen next. It's a peaceful quiet.

It occurs to me that many, if not most, of those in my audience may already have no recollection of what happened during the previous hour. When training new employees, I often mention that some individuals with short-term memory loss are unable to remember back more than three seconds. At least fifteen have elapsed since the end of our activity. I feel sad thinking the experience of the program may have already dissolved into thin air for many of those present.

Then Hal, sitting in the second row, turns to his friend Carmela and comments, "I like it here, don't you?"

Though not directed to me, I took Hal's remark as an unexpected compliment. He enjoyed the program, even if he couldn't recall anything about it afterward. Still, it left him with the sense that this space, this place, was a positive one.

Hal's words were a gift, reinforcing that engagement is meaningful for individuals when an experience captures their full attention, making dementia-related challenges irrelevant. A person is drawn into the moment and remains engaged in a relaxed and peaceful manner. Singing, costumes and raucous laughter may be involved, or maybe there's poetry, meditation and quiet conversation.

> Engagement is meaningful for individuals when an experience captures their full attention, making dementia-related challenges irrelevant.

No matter the activity, if it captivates attention, imagination and heart, people feel safe and are happy to remain in the room. They do not fret about getting home, whether the kids have been fed, or where their mother has gone. The space created is a haven where individuals can enjoy being right where they are, participating in what is happening now.

Evelyn and Hal taught me what is required when caring for people living with dementia. My role and goal became clear: to create experiences for our memory care community members in which connection, joy, fun and thriving mattered more than anyone's dementia-related deficits.

Throughout my work, I found it helpful to become comfortable with the unexpected.

Unusual Challenges

God bless me from a challenge!
—William Shakespeare, *Much Ado about Nothing*, act 5, sc. 1

Marlene

Marlene has developed a new habit. It is shocking to see one of our most beautiful and intelligent community members sticking her fingers in her mouth and flinging her saliva at the wall whenever it suits her.

We manage this, to some degree, by giving her gum to chew. We do our best to ensure she has a paper cup in her hand and remind her to spit into it at critical times. It's tricky, though, for a team member to be present at every single one of those moments.

That surprising lack of inhibition and decorum from Marlene was indeed a challenge. However, I've learned most surprises presented by people living with dementia are amusing, delightful or illuminating. Even if unwelcome, they prove instructive.

Sheila

Sheila talked at a furious pace in super-long sentences. Energetic, feisty and younger than most members of our assisted living community, her delightful Irish accent and easy laughter made her a breath of fresh air.

Not long after moving in, Sheila ordered a delivery of several boxes of liquor. She was diagnosed with Wernicke-Korsakoff syndrome, a type of dementia often associated with alcoholism. Her family was notified, the bottles were returned, and her means of ordering liquor was cut off. Sheila accepted the lack of easy access to alcohol without fuss, but after a while, curious things began to happen.

> On the third floor, where Sheila lives, items left inside unlocked apartments and decorations placed outside people's doors are disappearing. Care team members note Sheila has more possessions in her apartment than she used to, and they report she tends to walk the halls a lot.
>
> As the resident services director, it falls to me to investigate. I find several missing items in Sheila's apartment when she is elsewhere playing cards.
>
> Sheila has a total lack of impulse control when she sees an object she likes and wants for herself, which is a trait associated with many types of dementia, including Korsakoff syndrome.
>
> A devoted Catholic, Sheila attends afternoon Mass in our chapel. After the service, the priest, Father John, stands outside the doorway to greet each person as they exit. Before taking his place, he removes his stole—an ornate garment that drapes across his shoulders and hangs down his chest. It

symbolizes his role in ministry and his responsibility to serve God's people. Father John treasures this stole not only for its symbolic meaning but also because it was specially made for him overseas.

The Mass has just concluded. As usual, Father John folds his stole over a nearby chair before stepping outside the chapel. He greets each parishioner as they depart, then returns to retrieve his stole, only to discover the chair empty. Despite an exhaustive search, it is nowhere to be found.

I am not the only one who suspects Sheila's involvement in this situation. When I find her in her apartment, I ask, "Sheila, have you seen Father John's stole anywhere? By any chance, did you happen to pick it up?"

"Absolutely not! What would I ever want with a stole?" Sheila scolds.

When she is busy elsewhere, I check her room, but to no avail.

Several weeks go by. Then, one afternoon, when the mailman opens all the assisted living mailboxes, he is surprised by a stole, folded up, neat as can be, in a mailbox—Sheila's. He brings it to the front desk.

When the receptionist gives it to me a little while later, I waste no time tracking Sheila down to say, "Sheila, look what the mailman found in your mailbox."

Without missing a beat, Sheila delivers one of her long, lightning-fast sentences—in a single breath. "Well, I found it one day draped over a chair, so I brought it to the front desk to give to the afternoon receptionist to return to Father John, but she said she was swamped and couldn't take it right away, so I put it there in my mailbox for safekeeping until I saw her again."

Despite what you may think, Sheila was not telling a straightforward lie. While I understood people living with Korsakoff syndrome often create inaccurate memories and insist they are true, this was my first encounter with this phenomenon, known as confabulation. With every fiber of her being, Sheila believed every word she spoke. Chastising or accusing her was useless. This was evidence of Korsakoff syndrome at work in her brain.

> In the spirit of crossing to her side of the street, I reply, "Well, thank you for keeping it safe, Sheila." Then, I return the precious stole to a much relieved and grateful priest.

Medical writer Lorenzo Lucchetti explains that confabulation refers to the unintended creation of false memories. Though this is one of many symptoms of dementia, it can result from any brain illness or injury. Confabulation occurs when people are trying to fill in gaps in memory and do so through fabrication. As a result, people living with dementia may say things that are untrue or inaccurate while being convinced they are telling the truth. [32]

> People living with dementia may say things that are untrue or inaccurate while being convinced they are telling the truth.

Mom

One time, when I was visiting Mom in Denver, she was rushed to the hospital in an ambulance. I don't remember the specifics of the medical issue, but I can't forget what happened when I joined her in the emergency room.

32 Lorenzo Lucchetti, "Understanding Confabulation in Dementia," *Medical News Today*, November 20, 2023, emeraldlakebooks.com/confabulation.

I enter Mom's exam room, where she has been left alone. She is disoriented and delirious. No wonder, given the chaotic, unfamiliar atmosphere, the pain she is experiencing, and I suspect, the drugs administered to calm her down. (I learned much later that Mom had been given a medication that should not have been dispensed to anyone with Parkinson's disease, which we did not know she had at the time. This incident served as the initial indication for that diagnosis.)

If meds are involved, they are backfiring. Mom is striding around the space without her walker, singing "Let Me Call You Sweetheart" at the top of her lungs in the angriest voice imaginable. It's comical, yet also weird and disturbing. I can't seem to get her attention or slow her down enough to provide any comfort. So I press the call button. After a while, a nurse appears and transfers Mom to a hospital room.

In those days, "Let Me Call You Sweetheart" was Mom's favorite song. During the sing-alongs we attended together, her face would brighten with recognition at the first familiar notes of that tune.

Reflecting on that hospital scene, which feels like a strange dream, I think Mom may have been trying to calm herself by singing that song. Although she could not control her angry tone or make herself feel less disoriented, her inner resilience kicked in. She summoned the melody she loved and trusted most—a valiant attempt to counterbalance her distress.

If I could replay my role in that scene, I would try singing along with Mom, almost matching her energy level, but without any anger in my voice, to see if doing this would validate the intensity of her feelings and help relieve her distress. Whether it worked or not, I'm sure her response would have taught me another lesson.

Unusual challenges are humbling. We often don't have a clue how best to soothe a person's angst, respond to beliefs we know are incorrect, or react to a demonstration of the loss of inhibition.

One time, in the middle of our monthly birthday party, Caroline, a lovely woman who lived in memory care, walked up to the young male guitar player who was entertaining the crowd in the big dining room while most of us were busy digging into cake. She stood right in front of him and lifted her blouse to reveal her bare breasts. Many titters from the audience ensued. To his credit, the musician kept singing and strumming his guitar. Someone on the care team quickly shuttled a smiling Caroline back to her apartment for a wardrobe adjustment.

It helps to remind ourselves in situations like these that a significant decline in inhibition and impulse control can be part of dementia for some individuals. Understanding that a person really could not have acted differently is a regular practice for those working in memory care.

When we accept someone's unconventional behavior, we open the doorway a bit wider to our own learning. Why waste time judging? Was Caroline hurting anybody? Sure, the musician was probably a bit embarrassed, but he handled it professionally. Caroline certainly got some joy out of it, so why not be happy for her?

Instead of judgment, it pays to become curious in unanticipated situations and to remind ourselves that people are not the sum of whatever they do that doesn't align with expected standards of decorum. These occurrences remind us how important it is to focus on the strengths and skills that people living with dementia retain.

Surprising Skills

I am amazed, and know not what to say.
—William Shakespeare, *A Midsummer Night's Dream*, act 3, sc. 2

Bea

Bea is a proud, sophisticated woman still residing in assisted living, though her short-term memory is fading. She cannot tell you which day it is or what she had for breakfast. While she stares at the schedule of daily activities and writes down things she means to attend, she often doesn't show up when they take place.

A coworker discovers Bea used to play the piano but hasn't touched one for decades. After dinner, she brings Bea into our now-deserted memory care dining room, where our portable keyboard is parked.

Though Bea insists she no longer plays, she can't resist sitting on the piano bench. My coworker makes herself scarce, leaving

Bea alone with the instrument. She plays haltingly at first. Then, step by step, the notes knit together, as though she has found the right train track in her brain to catch a ride on.

The sound becomes effortless and haunting. For a full half hour, the lilting, romantic trills of classical music waft from the dining room into the nearby lobby. Bea's playing spans the keyboard, commanding and complex. Her touch is light, yet she communicates the majestic beauty of the composition.

Bea's passion for the piano had not deserted her. What a testament to the power of muscle memory and the strength of our brain's attachment to pastimes that bring us pleasure—even rapture. How sad that the social stigma and shame that often surround cognitive decline seem to encourage people to talk themselves into an "Oh, I can't do that anymore" mindset. This mode of thinking creates unnecessary embarrassment and grief for the individual.

As carers of those living with dementia, it falls to us to provide opportunities that will spark memories, awaken skills, and even surprise our charges with their retained prowess. In this effort, we remind people of a precious part of their identity that deserves to be honored.

Sarah

Sarah, an intelligent and animated woman, appears younger than most of our participants. She is involved in another group project that Jeanie, Zoë and I are in charge of, again engaging individuals living with dementia around the theme of love.

During our first session, I give a brief introduction to Shakespeare, for which I dust off parts of my Shakespearience program.

When I finish, Sarah is the first to comment. "Shakespeare!" she says with feigned disgust. "He never calls… He never writes!" Her comic timing and wit are a delight.

I was warned long ago to avoid using sarcasm around those in memory care, because they "might not understand" that type of humor, take it the wrong way, or feel offended. Yet here was a person living with dementia making a funny, sarcastic comment worthy of Dorothy Parker, the renowned American poet, critic and satirist.

Remain open to discovering exceptions to rules and generalizations.

While it is indeed good practice to avoid sarcasm around those experiencing dementia, it's important to remain open to discovering exceptions to rules and generalizations.

Every individual living with dementia is unique, and there are multiple causes and types of cognitive decline. One's personality may or may not remain consistent as it progresses. We should never make assumptions about a person's abilities based on the fact that they have a dementia-related diagnosis.

No doubt, winning a laugh from a good-sized audience made a meaningful difference to Sarah. Always be looking for opportunities to provide people experiencing dementia with whatever gives them an effective boost in mood or a sense of self-worth, a feeling that, "Hey, someone sees, appreciates and cares about me." It might consist of offering a compliment, singing their favorite song, taking a stroll together, seeking their advice, asking questions about things they love to talk about, sharing a hug (assuming permission has been granted), or simply enjoying a laugh together.

Gloria and Others

I wasn't sure whether an activity called "Learn a Little Shakespeare" would be well received in our memory care community, but I decided to give it a shot, betting that the several former English teachers in our group might enjoy it.

I write three lines from Romeo and Juliet's balcony scene in block letters on the whiteboard and read the first line aloud: "My bounty is as boundless as the sea."

I ask the group which word they think is the most important, that is, the one that best expresses the line's meaning. Their unanimous choice is "boundless." At drama school, we were encouraged to emphasize the most important word in a line when making sense of one of Shakespeare's verses.

I erase "boundless" and replace it with a blank line. I read back the remaining words. When I come to the blank, I ask the group to fill in what's missing. I am pleasantly surprised when, without hesitation, most of them say "boundless." The experiment is working.

We discuss every line in order. When asked to pick the most important word, most people choose the same one I would.

The process continues with the group picking out the second most important word in each line, and me replacing it with another blank. Then, I read what's still on the board and have them fill in the blanks.

We continue this process until the board has only blanks and a few punctuation marks. As I point to each one, we recite the missing word together. Of course, there are variations in how many of them individuals remember, but these folks do remarkable work with this brain exercise, despite living with dementia.

When I revisit this activity a month later, I begin with the same quote from Romeo and Juliet. I am surprised as well as tickled when Gloria (who isn't one of the former English teachers) remembers most of the words from four weeks earlier.

It was a gamble to try a Shakespeare-based activity in memory care. I wasn't sure whether people would be interested. However, even though the number of attendees was not large, those who came were eager to participate.

I do recommend planning something completely different from time to time, since new experiences are so beneficial for our brain cells. Another unusual event I have scheduled is a drumming circle. I was thrilled to observe how deeply captivating and soothing the session was for those living with dementia. If you work in memory care and have never brought in someone to lead one, please consider doing so. It's a way for many people to participate. For those of you who are carers at home, I encourage you to set your loved one up with a drum or a pot or pan and let them play too, with or without music.

Janine

Janine grew up in the United Kingdom. With her English accent, ready smile, and powerful speaking voice, she is the star of the Shakespeare portion of our Shakespeare, Poetry and Music project. She is comfortable reciting the Bard, and her diction is perfect. It is a true pleasure to listen to her delivery, which is energetic, confident and free of artifice.

I cue Janine with, "O Romeo, Romeo…" expecting her to chime in with, "Wherefore art thou, Romeo?" Instead, Janine replies, "Lend me your ears. I come to bury Caesar, not to praise him. The evil that men do lives after them; the good

> is oft interred with their bones." With an ominous tone, she continues. "So let it be with Caesar."
>
> Ignoring the jump to another play, everyone applauds Janine's expertise, and she beams. I swear, she recites Shakespeare better than many professional actors I've seen.

Janine entered hospice care several months after our project ended. I visited her on one of her last days. She was resting, lying on her side, and whispering. I couldn't make out anything she was saying. Before taking my leave, I spoke softly into her ear, repeating the snippets of Shakespeare I'd heard her deliver with poise and grace.

Just as Janine's skill with Shakespeare was inspiring to me, I encourage you to think about who in your care has surprised you with abilities you didn't know they possessed. Have you found ways to explore, celebrate and remind them of their skills and interests? Have they traveled to places others in your community or circle might be happy to hear about? Do they say things occasionally that are worth writing down and remembering? Keeping a journal for that purpose may come in handy later on. I wasn't at Janine's memorial service, but I hope a quote or two from Shakespeare was part of it.

Linda

> Linda has lived in our memory care community for several years now. She is struggling with depression and physical difficulties as dementia progresses.
>
> Her husband, Rick, hopes she will thrive in the smaller community to which he has decided to move her. I agree that a more home-like environment will better suit her needs.

To prevent any anxiety that might arise for Linda, Rick has let us know he will not tell her in advance about the move. Our care team understands that we should not mention the plan to Linda.

It's moving day, but she still doesn't know it. Early in the morning, before breakfast, Linda comes to my office, as she frequently does. Instead of sitting down, she lingers in the doorway while we chat. She is often wistful, and today is no exception.

Before leaving, Linda steadies her gaze on mine and says, "Have a nice life."

I hug her and wish her the same. With her artistic and spiritual sensitivity, I believe she feels the changing tide.

I was truly amazed and inspired by all the women in this chapter. They showed me how passionate people living with dementia can be. Bea so loved revisiting the piano, Sarah delighted in sharing her comic side and singing talent, Gloria was rightfully proud of her brain in the Shakespeare activity, Janine was so proficient speaking the Bard, and Linda possessed such gentleness and longing.

When we hear the word *dementia*, do most people usually think about how clever, zealous, smart, gifted and sensitive individuals living with it can be? We do them a serious disservice if we don't. Why deny ourselves the opportunity to appreciate what they have to reveal about themselves, which can be as delightful as it may be unexpected?

The women featured in this chapter, along with other individuals who wowed me with surprising skills, taught me that zest for life, precious memories, and impressive talents belong to all human beings, right alongside our quirks, foibles, mistakes and cognitive challenges. We must always remain curious about an individual's earlier accomplishments.

I recall learning that one brilliant gentleman who spent most of his time in his apartment was a career scientist. During World War II, he was an expert on the use of infrared photography. A very feisty woman had proudly served as a WAC, a member of the Women's Army Corps. Many people revealed their charming (or quirky) sense of humor. Others were exceptionally quiet souls, even-keeled, thoughtful and kind. And there were always some extroverts—perpetually chatty, full of funny stories, and gung ho to join whatever was going on.

People often enjoyed showing me their various collections, hobbies and interests inside their apartments, including tennis trophies, hand-crocheted doilies, and a large collection of exquisite dolls.

In a memory care community, there's always something in an individual's personal space begging to be asked about. These items are valuable clues. Find opportunities to talk with the person or their family to learn more regarding what is precious to them and whether they might enjoy sharing their hobby or passion with others.

It is a mistake to think that the condition of dementia could define or erase the worth of someone's existence. The more we celebrate the talents, skills, interests, experiences and attributes of individuals—including the capacity to feel and to express love—the healthier and happier they will remain in our care.

Expressions of Love

And when Love speaks, the voice of all the gods
Makes heaven drowsy with the harmony.

—William Shakespeare, *Love's Labour's Lost*, act 4, sc. 3

Lawrence

Lawrence must be sleeping, as usual. His eyes are closed, and his chin rests on his chest.

Two colleagues and I are using Shakespeare, poetry and music to engage a group of twenty people in various phases of dementia. We're focusing on the theme of love to inspire insights and stimulate memories.

"Where is love?" asks Zoë Bird, Director of the Alzheimer's Poetry Project Minnesota.

Jeanie Brindley-Barnett of the MacPhail Center for Music tinkles the piano keys with the opening notes of the song "Where Is Love?" from the Broadway musical *Oliver!*

A woman in our assembled group answers the question. "Well, it has to be somewhere. You have to be able to find it."

"You have to be able to find it," repeats Zoë as I write that phrase down on a giant whiteboard. "Where do you find it?" Zoë asks the group.

Suddenly, Lawrence perks up. After lifting his head, he takes a deep breath and answers with confidence, "Love is at first sight."

"Love is at first sight," repeats Zoë. "Do you want to say more about that?"

Lawrence sure does. He takes another large breath. "Well, I found love very easily. I was working at Armors and living at the YMCA. This young fella comes up to me and says, 'Say, you were in the Army, and I heard you was a cook. Well, I live upstairs and don't know how to boil water.' I said, 'Well, I live at the YMCA and could probably teach you how to cook a little bit.' Then, here comes a girl down the steps. Wha-aat a girl! 'How does a person get into this room?' I ask. She says, 'You know what, I used to live up there. I'll run up and get you a key, and you can keep it because I forgot to give it back.'" Lawrence lets out a profound sigh.

"Was that the beginning?" asks Jeanie with a knowing smile. There's a brief pause.

"You know what? I married her!" Lawrence produces an even bigger sigh and repeats, "What a girl." He straightens himself up and proclaims with great energy, "Love at first sight. Love at first sight. Love at first sight!"

Remembering how Lawrence repeated that phrase three times with such intensity still moves me to tears years later. His memory of his first encounter with his future wife was a stunning affirmation of the depth of passion we carry right along with us into older age, dementia be damned.

It is natural for humans to want to remember and discuss the experiences that have shaped our lives and given them meaning.

Lawrence's detailed recitation of their meeting taught me never to assume someone is sleeping, bored or inattentive because their eyes are closed. His response to the music and Zoë's gentle prompts was a moving example of how people with dementia can be restored to a sense of self through meaningful interaction, music and fond memories.

It is natural for humans to want to remember and discuss the experiences that have shaped our lives and given them meaning. It was fortunate Lawrence's story was captured on film and is part of the documentary, *From the Valley of the Heart*, produced by Ebenezer Senior Living and featuring the collaboration I initiated with two other professional teaching artists.[33]

Some time later, it may have been the same day when he shared about meeting his future wife, the usually sleepy Lawrence amazed us again with his willingness to take on a character in a short scene from Shakespeare's *A Midsummer Night's Dream*. He played Bottom, an unsophisticated weaver by trade, who is transformed into a donkey by the mischievous fairy Puck. Lawrence's "hee-haws" were legendary—long and loud after a substantial inhale. His performance induced many giggles from all assembled. I think sharing his love story must have opened up something affirming and strengthening for Lawrence!

33 Ebenezer, "From The Valley of the Heart," YouTube video, posted January 8, 2019, emeraldlakebooks.com/ebenezerdoc.

Mom

I remember one of the last times I saw Mom.

> Mom emerges from her room, pushing her walker as I approach her in the hallway. A few months have passed since my last visit. I've been told she isn't speaking much these days, and it occurs to me she may not remember my name. When I get close, Mom stops in her tracks and cocks her head, fixing her gaze on mine. She doesn't say a word, but after several seconds, her eyes soften. The love emanating from them is unmistakable and overpowering.

Mom gave me a wonderful gift with that look. Her eyes told me she knew I was someone she loved. Her gaze assured me love doesn't depend on words exchanged or understood, on whether people know your name or say what you expect to hear. When love is present, we feel it.

In that moment, I received additional proof that individuals living with dementia do not lose the ability to feel, give and receive love. There is still a person in there with whom we can connect.

Defiance and Conviction

Take my defiance!

—William Shakespeare, *Measure for Measure*, act 3, sc. 1

Agatha

When I started working in dementia care, Agatha was the first person to move into our brand-new memory care community. She arrived on foot via the long hallway that attached it to the independent living side of our building.

Agatha established herself in her new environment as quite a character. Small in stature, she was self-sufficient, stubborn and prickly-never shy about speaking her mind. No one knew why, but every time she saw Jill, our cheerful, easygoing campus administrator, Agatha would say, with a deadpan expression, "Well, look who you run into when you don't have a shotgun!" Agatha was hilarious, with an edge. I could imagine that back in the day, on the farm, she had known how to handle a gun.

After a decade in memory care, Agatha's increasing needs resulted in her transfer to a skilled nursing center. At 101 years old, she was a bona fide legend to all who loved her, and we were saddened to see her go.

It's been a few weeks since Agatha moved out. I miss her and have arranged to drop by her new place for a visit. She is in a good mood and is sharp and chatty, as usual. She appears unfazed by the change in setting, despite the dramatic downgrade in comfort and privacy. Instead of an apartment or a room, she has a bed and several movable partitions in a spacious open area with a high ceiling.

Halfway through our visit, a nurse barges in and attempts to give Agatha a pill. She responds with a long and boisterous scream, "No-o!"

In all my years working in memory care, I never heard Agatha scream.

The nurse tries harder to get the medicine into Agatha's mouth. Guess how well this goes over? She screams even louder, and the nurse slinks away in defeat.

Agatha turns to me, eyes shining. With perfect calm, she says in her gruff, throaty voice, "You can't let 'em win every time." She punctuates this with a broad grin.

I laugh out loud. I'm proud of her. She is going to be fine.

Agatha's response confirmed the critical importance of a respectful, compassionate approach. People who are living with dementia won't "let 'em win" if they're treated in a bossy, forceful, "my way or the highway" manner that fails to connect with them first. This lesson from Agatha serves as a key reminder of the dramatic difference the tone of our approach can make.

Christine

Christine, a petite woman prone to erratic moods, recently transitioned to memory care and is unhappy with the change. Accustomed to independence in assisted living, she is having a hard time adjusting to her new caregivers. In particular, she is uncomfortable accepting help from people who are not White.

Today, Oroni, who is from Africa, is assigned to Christine. Oroni goes into Christine's room to help her dress, but before they begin, Christine screams at Oroni to get out. Her tirade includes swearing and use of the N-word.

It's unfortunate I am not trained in delivering personal care and cannot take Oroni's place. As Christine's tantrum escalates over several minutes, I find our medication assistant, Awa, the only other attendant available on the floor. I ask her if she will try to help Christine. Because Awa, who is Gambian, also has dark skin, I am not at all confident this "change of face" strategy will prove more effective than Oroni's attempt.

Awa, bless her, is willing. After Oroni leaves, Awa enters Christine's apartment. With supreme calm, confidence and vocal warmth, she announces, "I'll help you, Christine. I'm not Black."

Lo and behold, Christine accepts her care.

I learned valuable lessons from Awa and Christine that day. It was wrong of me to assume Christine wouldn't accept help from another Black caregiver. I underestimated Awa's ability to achieve a different outcome. She brought courage and sensitivity to a fraught situation. Her creativity in choosing an unconventional tactic, despite the strong chance it might fail, was extraordinary. Christine couldn't help but be comforted by Awa's gentle approach and beautiful smile. Exhaustion resulting from her continued outburst may also have contributed to Christine's willingness to accept Awa's care.

This episode showed me that when you don't know how to help someone living with dementia who is upset or distressed, it pays to stay calm , manage your tone of voice and, like Awa, think outside the box.

While it can be complicated to work with people when their moods or beliefs are challenging, keep in mind that these situations are golden opportunities to learn what works and what doesn't. Sometimes people living with dementia believe they need to find their car, get to work, or pick up the kids. It may be tricky to convince them that all is as it should be. However, acknowledging their worry and promising to "talk to the manager" about, say, where their car might be parked, can give some measure of solace. Saying, "If I were you, I would feel the same way," to acknowledge their concern about their children, or admiring their sense of responsibility about being on time, may help calm the person down a notch. "Tell me more about your job" can be an effective distraction if you ask a lot of questions about it. I've seen some people let go of obsessing about getting to work when simply told they have the day off today. If necessary, having a family member corroborate this over the phone can be helpful, as well as distracting. What is most important for your success in managing these tough situations is that you communicate clearly that you are on the person's side, appreciate their worry, and understand their feelings.

> When you don't know how to help someone living with dementia who is upset or distressed, it pays to stay calm.

Thankfully, most of the individuals I cared for, once they became acclimated to their new community, were more often funny and playful than they were worried, incorrigible or defiant.

Personality and Playfulness

Play with your fancies
—William Shakespeare, *Henry V*, act 3, prologue

Dottie

We are accustomed to hearing Dottie call "Whoo-hoo" from inside her apartment whenever she needs assistance. Today, Dottie is whoo-hooing loud and clear in the hallway. I'm nearby and hurry to her side to see if I can help with anything.

"Oh no," is Dottie's amiable reply. "I'm just letting off steam." Smiling from ear to ear, she continues to chug along, pushing her walker and whoo-hooing to her heart's content.

The next time I see Dottie's son, a frequent visitor, I ask him, "Has Dottie always been so good-natured and fun?"

In all seriousness, he answers, "Oh no! She was a real grump."

Well, I think to myself, *that's one point for dementia, for sure.*

The Dottie I knew was a riot. Supremely playful, she was also a devout Catholic who loved reciting this sweet prayer:

Angel of God,
my guardian dear,
To whom His love
commits me here,
Ever this day
be at my side,
To light and guard,
To rule and guide.

Fred

Fred always looks neat and put together in his gray suit and tie. He is one of the most congenial people I have ever met. He will shake your hand, smile and introduce himself with his first and last name every time he sees you, as though you have never met before.

Fred worked in a top-secret government position, and he must have been exceptional. He exudes trustworthiness. Despite the suit and tie, Fred seems more like a beloved grade school teacher, the friendliest mailman ever, or a guy who ran a small neighborhood business. You never know.

Marlene

One of my favorite activities came from *The Best Friends Book of Alzheimer's Activities*.[34] I heard the coauthor of this guide, David

34 Virginia Bell, David Troxel, Tonya M. Cox, and Robin Hamon, *The Best Friends Book of Alzheimer's Activities, Volume 1* (Baltimore, MD: Health Professions Press, 2014), 195, "Mona Lisa and the Art of Good Alzheimer's Care."

Troxel, present at a conference many years ago. He described a fun activity involving the *Mona Lisa*, and I was eager to try it out.

David recommended getting a large poster of the *Mona Lisa*, but we didn't need one once I discovered Val, one of our memory care ladies, had a large throw blanket in her apartment with an image of the famous painting. She was happy to let me borrow this for our activity.

On the day, I tape Val's blanket to our whiteboard. I have a bunch of scarves and fabric pieces ready to go, and a recording of Nat King Cole singing "Mona Lisa."

The activity begins with everyone humming or singing along with Nat to that familiar tune. Then, I invite them to take turns sitting in front of the blanket backdrop to pose as Mona Lisa. I drape scarves and fabric around each person's head and shoulders to suggest Mona Lisa's sixteenth-century garb and encourage them all to imitate the famous and enigmatic Mona Lisa smile.

These women are eager to play. Everyone giggles during a spirited discussion of various possibilities regarding what or who Mona Lisa is thinking about. I photograph each person as they pose and smile.

When it's Marlene's turn, she displays her dramatic flair with enthusiasm. Her improvised monologue of Mona Lisa's thoughts about Leonardo, punctuated by exaggerated facial expressions, draws us all into a playful mood. Although it borders on the risqué, everyone enjoys this to the hilt.

I highly recommend providing activities for those living with dementia that allow them to both relax and let their creative imaginations run wild. Creativity does not disappear simply because someone reaches a certain age or begins living with dementia.

Ida

I'm bringing Ida down to the first floor for an activity. She is out of sorts, grumbling as I wheel her onto the elevator. I kneel at her eye level to see if I can cheer her up.

"Well, Ida, you know what they say—when life hands ya lemons, whaddaya supposed to do?"

Ida stares at me, still cross, as I await her answer. Then, her grumpy visage morphs into that of a mischievous elf as she exclaims, "Make whoopee!"

We are both laughing loud enough to draw attention as the elevator doors open. I believe I am more cheered than she is.

Eleanor

Eleanor is vibrant and movie-star pretty. Her enormous blue eyes remind me of the irrepressible actress Carol Channing. Proud of her service in the Women's Army Corps during World War II, Eleanor cherishes the time she lived in New York City. She speaks with fondness of the "good old days" when she and the "gals" would frequent bars to stir up some fun. She longs for her late husband and misses him "every single day." Eleanor is articulate, thoughtful and aware of her cognitive decline, which to me is almost invisible.

I've seated our large group of ladies, Eleanor included, in a circle to reminisce about aprons. Three Friends InDeed volunteers are here to help. It's their first experience in memory care. One volunteer, Ethel, is excited to share the apron her mother made for her, which she brought along.

A wicker basket contains a hefty pile of wrinkled aprons I found at a secondhand store. We pass these around, try them on, discuss which ones we like and which we don't, decide if any might appeal to our mothers, and consider various occasions when we might choose to wear this one or that one.

Sunlight streams through the windows on this chilly February afternoon. Everyone is delighted to touch, try on, and discuss the collection of old aprons.

Next, Ethel unpacks the prized yellow-checked apron her mother sewed. It's been ironed, wrapped in tissue paper, and stored with care in a box. After she shows it around the circle for all to admire, Ethel surprises me by grabbing a plastic bag from under her chair and pulling out another apron. She presents this one to me as a gift. It's bright pink with an enormous red heart on it. Of course, I am obliged to model my new apron for the group.

As I tie the sash, Eleanor blurts out, loud and clear enough for anyone in the room with hearing difficulties to understand, "Oh! Oh! Wear that on Valentine's Day when you make dinner for your husband. Wear that and nothing else. Been there, done that!"

The entire room erupts with robust giggles and guffaws, which makes us laugh even more. Volunteers, women living with dementia, and I are all helpless with laughter, like thirteen-year-olds at a slumber party. We keep laughing for five whole minutes.

I am forever grateful to Eleanor for her sense of humor—and her lack of impulse control, which may have contributed to her comment. My volunteers learned firsthand, in a more effective way than I could ever explain, that people living with dementia are, above all, people. They are as capable of sharing raucous laughter with friends as anyone else. Dementia posed no challenges while we were involved with aprons and giggling with abandon.

People living with dementia are, above all, people.

As caregivers, it is important to have fun and provide opportunities to deliver unbridled enjoyment to those you are responsible for. Remember, people experiencing dementia are losing skills in the reverse order in which they were gained while growing up. Once the abilities learned in adulthood begin to fade, they move into the middle stage of dementia. At this point, individuals may remind you more of the teenagers you've known, raised or been. For example, you might notice more disorganization in their thoughts and in their rooms, along with more frequent emotional highs and lows. In addition, these folks often show increased interest in socializing with others and simply having a good time, including listening to or telling jokes. And if there's a sexual innuendo to be shared there, so much the better!

Living Well with Dementia While Maintaining Integrity

I love long life better than figs.

—William Shakespeare, *Antony and Cleopatra*, act 1, sc. 2

Barney

"Go home. Get your affairs in order. There's no cure."

Imagine hearing those words from a doctor after receiving a diagnosis of Alzheimer's disease or any other form of dementia. Or hearing "Come back when she can't feed herself." That comment was delivered to the husband of a woman who was being diagnosed. Over the course of the appointment, the doctor spoke directly to him—not at all to his patient.

At the first Dementia Action Alliance (DAA) conference I attended in 2017, I was shaken and moved by the panel participants—individuals living with dementia and their partners—who shared their appalling experiences of receiving the initial diagnosis. The DAA is an organization dedicated to supporting people seeking to live well with dementia. I was grateful to witness the strength and resolve that the panelists were capable of. I learned they were defying stereotypes at every turn.

Two years later, at the next conference, several of the same individuals spoke onstage again, along with others living with dementia. The people I had seen the first time did not seem to have progressed much, if at all, in terms of the severity of their condition. They remained as articulate, energized and committed as ever, driven by the purpose of sharing their experiences and their adaptation and compensation strategies with others.

Many of those involved with DAA travel in the USA and overseas to speak at conferences or consult with other organizations. How different these individuals are from those I knew when I first worked in a memory care community! I imagine each person I cared for back then may well have received a diagnosis of dementia that felt like a death sentence, leaving them in despair.

At the 2022 DAA conference, I met Barney and his partner, Vicki. At the trade show, they displayed Twiddle samples.[35] These activity/comfort aids are designed to help people of all ages with various sensory-related conditions. Twiddle muffs are soft and outfitted with beads and other things that invite touch and manipulation. Twiddles are useful for those living with mid-to-late-stage dementia and for children on the autism spectrum. Barney and Vicki also had AdaptiWraps on display. These easy-to-put-on sweaters are helpful for elders with mobility or cognitive issues. We chatted briefly, and Barney and Vicki were so kind as to give me an AdaptiWrap for anyone I knew who might benefit from it. After the conference, they extended the generous offer of free samples of both Twiddles and AdaptiWraps to ten Ebenezer care communities.

It wasn't until several months later, while paging through a publication from DAA titled *Pathways to Well-Being with*

35 Find more information about Twiddles and related comfort products at 4twiddles.com.

Dementia, that I was surprised to find a photo of Barney and a page of insights he had contributed to this manual. Until that moment, I did not know he was living with a dementia-related diagnosis.

I saw Barney and Vicki again at a local industry trade show the following year. I wanted to learn more about his situation and what had been most helpful to him. We arranged a Zoom meeting.

I learned that in 2019, Barney began to experience concerning tremors and hallucinations that prompted him to see a neurologist. His brain scan showed signs of Lewy body dementia. He was told to expect "three years that would be fairly normal, three years of challenges, then three years of absolute hell."

The prediction of "challenges" did not come to pass. Five years after his initial diagnosis, Barney was doing great. From time to time, he experienced mild Parkinsonian symptoms, but nothing too debilitating. His hallucinations subsided, and his cognitive abilities were pronounced "remarkable" by his doctor. Although his condition was previously thought to be Lewy body dementia, his neurologist reconsidered his earlier assessment and concluded that the symptoms fell within the range of mild cognitive impairment, also known as MCI.

Barney's turnaround is hopeful and inspiring. He attributes his improvement to his three-times-a-week sessions of Rock Steady Boxing. He includes tennis and dancing in his exercise regimen. Barney, a former business executive, served on the Advisory Board for DAA for a time and now consults with dementia trainer Teepa Snow's organization, sometimes presenting alongside her at events.

> If one is diagnosed with dementia, the key is to "own your diagnostic journey."

I was struck by the final insight Barney shared in our conversation. He said that if one is diagnosed with dementia, the key is to "own your diagnostic journey." For Barney, this means a wholehearted acceptance of his diagnosis and the emotions it provokes. This allowed him to move forward with power and clarity, managing the path ahead and making new choices. "Owning his journey" is how Barney managed to accomplish an impressive improvement. I'm grateful for his willingness to share his success, and I plan to take his advice to heart if I ever need it.

Rich

I almost forgot to mention Rich. Dementia is not top of mind when I think about him. He is one of my closest male friends and a funny, delightful person. There is frequent laughter when I get together with him and his charming life partner, Vic, who has also become a dear friend.

Rich and I met decades ago, when he owned a film production company. Years later, he directed the documentary I mentioned earlier, *From the Valley of the Heart*, which Ebenezer Senior Living produced. Vic put her considerable organizational skills into helping us see the project through to completion after Rich experienced a stroke.

Rich has lived with the repercussions of that event and was diagnosed with vascular dementia. Although he deals with aphasia, word-finding difficulties, memory issues, and confusion, his sense of humor, enjoyment of life, and passion for movies, theater and music remain intact.

Despite the challenges his brain presents, he comes across as himself, through and through. Rich has written and performed in a play about his stroke experience and enjoys meeting with an aphasia group. Playing music and socializing with friends are essential pastimes. Vic provides exceptional ongoing support for him and is always on the lookout for learning, entertainment and travel experiences for them to enjoy together.

Barney and Rich have taught me to no longer feel surprised by people who are living well with a dementia-related diagnosis. They often surprise you with what they have accomplished.

Julia

Integrity. That word has to do with truth and honesty, ideals that can get murky in dementia care as we strive to validate feelings and respect how an individual living with dementia sees and understands their world. When I was first asked to speak at a special event and share an example of integrity observed in eldercare, Julia was the first person who came to mind. But to tell the truth—ahem—I was not a hundred percent sure I could spin her story into a perfect fit for the value of integrity.

In dementia care, integrity is related to honoring and celebrating each person's core identity, connecting with their passions, skills, accomplishments and dreams.

I heard that a British opera singer had moved into one of our memory care sites. I was excited to meet her and hoped to get her interested in the Shakespeare, Poetry and Music project I would be co-leading at this community.

Several weeks before the project began, Julia and I were introduced as she lay in bed. I was thrilled to listen to her talk about her operatic career, touring abroad, and performing in Prague and other European capitals. Her eyes shone with pride as she shared how overjoyed she had been to sing with Pavarotti.

Resting her head on a pillow during the entirety of our conversation, Julia was cheerful, hospitable and animated. She loved reminiscing about her performances. She had sung onstage in musicals too. When I asked her what roles she played, she replied in her charming Northern English accent, "Ai played Laurie in *Oklahoma!* But now, muh voice isn't wha it used ta be, and Ai really down't sing mooch anymoh."

I couldn't wait for Julia to attend our Friday sessions. She hadn't made it to the last two, but she felt well enough to come to the next one, which focused on music. Bright-eyed and engaged throughout, Julia was often the first person to respond when my colleague Jeanie asked the group a music-related question.

Near the end of the hour, Jeanie tinkled the opening notes of "People Will Say We're in Love," the famous love duet from the musical *Oklahoma!* She invited Julia to sing the song with her. Julia didn't hesitate, even though she sounded creaky and warbling at first; she poured her whole heart into the effort. As Julia gained confidence, Jeanie backed off. By the time Julia hit the high notes near the end of the song, her voice was soaring across the room, pure and free. Everyone present could well imagine the singer she used to be. Memory care community members and resident assistants clapped and cheered when the tune finished. I glanced at Jeanie and saw tears sliding down her face, just like mine.

I remember thinking, as far as I was concerned, our project was already a success—one person had a chance to share her talent in front of a group and was appreciated with heartfelt applause.

Julia attended one other session, but after the first few minutes, she felt unwell and was taken back to her apartment to rest. Her health continued to deteriorate, and she passed away a few months later.

It's been a month since Julia died. I'm waiting for her daughter, Emily, to arrive at the coffee shop. Curious to hear more about Julia's career, I'm hoping Emily can loan me some recordings and playbills to incorporate into the documentary we're making about our project. I regret that the film crew was not on site on the day Julia sang.

Emily arrives. After some chit-chat and a few sips of coffee, I explain why I had asked her to meet with me. She hesitates, then breaks the news to me that Julia's memory, once she started living with dementia, had… expanded the extent of her career.

In fact, Julia had not toured the capitals of Europe. She hadn't ever met or sung with Pavarotti. Though she'd performed with a few nonprofessional light opera companies, she never did any professional work. Julia had indeed played Laurie in *Oklahoma!*—at a community theater—but the impressive career she described in grand detail to me and many others existed only in her imagination, fueled by dementia.

I must admit, I am shocked and disillusioned to learn all this. However, my next thought is, "Wow. Good for her." Given the options, who wouldn't welcome the type of memory loss that lets you remember your fondest dreams and expectations as reality?

I believe there's integrity to be found in what Julia's brain concocted for her. If integrity is defined as the quality or state of being complete or undivided, given that her mind was in harmony with her memory and aspirations, she was fully at peace with herself. What could be better than living our dreams—even if that occurs, unbeknownst to us, solely in our imagination?

The Ultimate Gift

A gift that heaven gives
—William Shakespeare, *Henry VIII*, act 1, sc. 1

Mom

I am at work when I receive a call from my sister with the news that Mom slipped away early this morning. Before her passing, she was given a warm bath and tucked back into bed by her favorite caregiver at her skilled care community.

Several hours after the call, I am on an airplane to Denver to join my sister and brother. Slumped in my seat, I attempt to absorb the reality of Mom being gone. I am deep in my raw grief. Relieved to have three seats to myself, a host of memories and emotions swirl inside me.

Mom was the heart and soul of our family. My siblings and I took inspiration from her kindness and care, while at times grappling with the strict judgments of our conscientious father.

Although he had an endearing, softer side—revealed through his wit and eloquence when delivering emotional toasts at family gatherings—it took time for each of his five children to truly appreciate him. In the meantime, Mom was more demonstrative, empathetic and emotionally present.

Mom sometimes laughed so hard at things Dad said that it brought her to tears. Then she'd exclaim, "Oh, Lordy!" and laugh some more. This expression tickled me and made me laugh too. Mom was steadfast in her devotion to, understanding of, and admiration for her husband, whom she had known well for most of their lives.

When I was forty-three, after being married—and miserable—for a decade, I called Mom to tell her I was getting a divorce. Her response was a testament to her awareness that I needed to figure out certain things for myself, no matter how long it took. She said, "Honey, I've been waiting for the call."

At forty-five, after two years of thinking nothing could feel more wonderful than being divorced, I married Phil. When we were in high school, Phil was one of my best friends and, for a few minutes (well, three weeks), my boyfriend. (It's a long story.)

Mom, at age eighty, attended our wedding. I remember her looking at Phil with the same smiling yet bewildered expression she sometimes wore in his presence when we were teenagers. Back then, he often joined us for dinner on Friday nights, ensuring my parents and I would have plenty of laughs around the kitchen table. Both Phil and my dad had deep, resonant voices, but the similarity ended there. While Mom might have had her doubts about Phil back then, I'm confident that when we got married decades later, she respected a love that had begun in high school.

Mom was an avid reader. I remember feeling aghast as a teenager when she spoke about how much she enjoyed reading Truman Capote's *In Cold Blood*, the true story of a set of gruesome murders committed in her home state of Kansas. Until I reached my forties, I didn't think I could handle opening that book. When I finally read it, I couldn't put it down. It was easy to understand why she loved it. Ten years later, I re-read it, and I might well do that again.

One time, while home from college, I was surprised to find a poster of "Desiderata" hanging near Mom's desk. This prose poem by Max Ehrmann was first published in 1927. It gained significant popularity during the 1970s and conveyed a spiritual message that, like Mom, I was drawn to.

"Desiderata"

This popular poem is packed with helpful, timeless advice. Here are a few lines that especially resonate with me:

> Go placidly amid the noise and the haste, and remember what peace there may be in silence.
>
> Nurture strength of spirit to shield you in sudden misfortune. But do not distress yourself with dark imaginings. Many fears are born of fatigue and loneliness.
>
> Beyond a wholesome discipline, be gentle with yourself. You are a child of the universe, no less than the trees and the stars; you have a right to be here.
>
> With all its sham, drudgery and broken dreams, it is still a beautiful world.

Mom taught me to sew and encouraged all my creative efforts. She gave me the option of not returning to the Saturday painting class I took when I was in third grade. The instructor had the nerve to fill in the background of my attempted pansies because I was taking "too much time" to replicate the details of each flower. I was too shy to confront her, but when I returned home that afternoon, I was as outraged as an introverted third grader could be by Mrs. Whatever-Her-Name-Was's hostile takeover of my painting. Mom came to my defense and phoned the teacher. There was no pressure from Mom for me to stay in the class, but I remained, despite the distrust I couldn't shake. I have respected my rather slow creative process ever since.

Mom adored my canary, Chipper, a poor replacement for a dog, the pet I had actually longed for. Chipper trilled his heart out whenever she vacuumed, which charmed her and won me over too. Through example, Mom taught me kindness, showed me how to persevere, get things done, help others, write thank-you notes, laugh and love—even through difficult times when one might feel lonely or unsure. She endured the trials of widowhood, Parkinson's disease and, of course, dementia. At one point, she faced a horrific and painful bout of shingles. As the years passed, she showed that people can become calmer with aging—which I am working on.

On the plane, I pull out the large manila envelope I had stuffed into my backpack before leaving the house. It's from an older cousin whom I haven't seen or heard from in several years, and it had come in the mail a minute before Phil drove me to the airport.

I open the envelope, which contains the latest issue of the local newspaper in Junction City, Kansas, Mom and Dad's hometown. There is no explanatory note from my cousin inside. I'm annoyed, having no idea why in the world she sent me this issue.

After scanning the first page, which isn't at all interesting, given my current emotional state, I have an impulse to shove the paper back into its envelope for good. But I change my mind. Sighing, I realize I might as well see what's happening in Junction City. I turn to the next page to discover an 8x10″ photograph of two high school students from an earlier era.

Breathless, I recognize the young lady: my mother-to-be. She is smiling, sitting on a decorative bench beside a handsome young man who is focused on inspecting the back of her right hand. A curtain hangs behind them. The caption beneath the photo informs me that this image captures a moment from a high school production of a play called "The Mummy and The Mumps."

The article reveals that the young man holding my mother's hand grew up to become a beloved doctor who practiced in Junction City. In his early nineties, he had just passed away, which explains why this full two-page tribute to him in the *Junction City Weekly Union* is now before my eyes.

I am astounded, not least because of the synchronicity of having this photo land in my lap on this particular day, but also because I never knew or even suspected Mom had performed onstage. Did I ever ask her if she had participated in school plays? No. I never even thought of inquiring. I am full of regret that I did not. It's baffling why she chose not to share that fact with me when I was involved in theater throughout high school, college and beyond.

What a mistake to assume my mother was too shy and quiet ever to perform. How insensitive of me, given that I identify as an introvert despite sporadic evidence to the contrary.

Another lesson from Mom—and what a tremendous gift. If I don't know this about her, how much am I missing about the people for whom I plan and carry out activities? I commit to learning more and not presuming I am aware of everything concerning what individuals living with dementia have done, or can or cannot do.

If not for my mom, I doubt I would have worked in dementia care. I would not possess the passion I have for this field, nor the insider knowledge of how dementia may challenge the person who is diagnosed with it, as well as their family members. I would not have the same drive to support creative engagement with individuals living with dementia, nor the motivation to ensure the care we provide is loving, empathetic and validating.

May you enjoy the gift of seeing people for who they truly are, as well as what they have done, and may they humble your assumptions when needed, bring you laughter, and stir your heart.

Expect More

For now sits Expectation in the air
—William Shakespeare, *Henry V*, act 2, prologue

Have you wondered whether your path in life will involve significant cognitive decline? You are not alone; I go there too, more than I care to admit. Life is so busy these days that we easily forget things and then worry about why we are forgetting. Our attention spans are so short now that it's hard not to see cognitive decline around every corner and wonder if it is coming to get us. Given that there are tests that can predict the likelihood of us one day living with dementia, you might find yourself wishing for a dementia vaccine or some other easy way to avoid a difficult diagnosis. (I provide a few suggestions in Appendix A on page 167 that may help.) A more realistic hope is that people around the world will become more aware of the increasing body of knowledge and resources available for preventing and managing significant cognitive decline.

I wonder… Can we do what it takes to "vaccinate" ourselves against the hopelessness, stigma and false assumptions people sometimes succumb to when interacting with those who live with dementia? Anne Basting, a visionary in the realm of creativity and dementia care and author of the book *Creative Care,* encourages us with the insight that joy and meaning can coexist even during the most challenging times of our lives.[36]

Let's stop underestimating people living with dementia and expecting less from them. Instead, let's strive to recognize and honor the humanity in each person and learn all we can from them.

If living with dementia becomes part of my journey, here's how I like to imagine it:

> My friends and family refuse to let dementia define me. Those who care for me understand that I still experience a range of emotions. Sometimes, I giggle with abandon. I can still be moved to tears.
>
> People place things in my hands that make me smile—objects or other items I can admire, touch, squeeze, smell or taste. They notice and calm my darker moods. I feel loved, appreciated and uplifted.
>
> Someone plays the music I love, they sing with me, and I sing to myself. I continue to paint and write (even if the marks I put on paper are not decipherable to others).
>
> Every part of my body that I can control gets practice moving. I often get outdoors, and I admire the beauty outside my window when I cannot.
>
> Regardless of whether I remember their names, I recall how different individuals make me feel. Deep down, I know who I have loved and still love, even if I cannot express that in words that make sense to anyone else. Dementia does not

36 Anne Basting, *Creative Care,* (New York: HarperOne, 2020), 4–5.

> diminish my desire to help, nor can it extinguish my passion for Shakespeare.
>
> My drive to connect, to give and receive affection, remains strong. My caregivers recognize that my spirit is intact. Rather than concentrating on deficits and losses as my dementia progresses, the people who care for me continue to explore my strengths, interests, heart and humor.
>
> If you happen to be among those who interact with me and perhaps others living with dementia, you are finding numerous ways to make a dramatic and positive difference in our lives. You feel the energy of the gift you give to yourself when you invest your time and apply your skills to serve others.
>
> Since you notice your instincts are often correct, your confidence grows along with your expanding toolbox. Best of all, you feel the remarkable joy of discovering what each person living with dementia has to teach you.

Sincere thanks for everything you have done and will do to look past dementia and learn from those in your care.

I invite you to check out the recommended reading on my website at lookpastdementia.com/resources to continue learning from those touched by dementia and from authors who share their discoveries and experiences.

The Light Ahead

[We] should notwithstanding join our lights together
And over-shine the earth

—William Shakespeare, *III Henry VI*, act 2, sc. 1

After more than three years of writing, reflecting and learning, I am thrilled the book is now in your hands. The next steps are up to you. How will this impact you and those in your life who are living with dementia?

I hope what sticks with you is that people living with dementia are still full-fledged human beings, doing their best despite challenges wrought by significant cognitive decline, and that a dementia diagnosis does not mean life is over. Joy, fun and meaningful relationships are not only possible but necessary for any person to thrive. If my book has reminded you of the benefits of being patient, using creativity, and always respecting the humanity of the individual, no matter how they are expressing themselves, I am pleased.

Even if you find yourself exhausted, grieving, uncertain, overwhelmed, discouraged or afraid of making a mistake, remind yourself: Of course you feel this way! (Validation is not only for those living with dementia.) Your role as caregiver, care partner, family member, or friend is not always easy. Everyone needs their emotions—happy or not—reflected through sharing, commiseration, venting or simply hearing and feeling that someone understands.

You may occasionally be caught off guard by a person's bad mood, sudden rage, or increased confusion. An approach you used successfully in the past may no longer work. This is normal and nothing to beat yourself up about. Instead, view this as an excellent twofold opportunity for validating whatever feelings are being communicated and changing your behavior accordingly. Try offering an apology: "I'm so sorry, George. I see that I've upset you. Let's start over. Tell me exactly how you'd like me to help, step by step."

I am most grateful for the depth of knowledge that twelve years working in dementia care provided. Interacting with Evelyn, Ida, Hal, Ollie and so many others became a daily practice of acceptance, friendship and love. After leaving that community to take on a dementia-focused educational role, I didn't fully realize how impactful the memories of those early experiences would continue to be until I realized I was getting close to the age of many of those in that collection of interesting souls. I felt how acutely I missed being with them. I loved the excitement of never knowing exactly what lessons each day might bring. There was so much to ponder, understand, enjoy and appreciate. I'm certain this work made me a more empathetic and emotionally available person.

I learned from those I served that relationships are vital, humanity is permanent, identity is fluid, love and joy are essential, purpose is fundamental to happiness, communication is not all about words, and dignity has nothing to do with one's age, looks or brain function. Dignity is a human right.

When my daughter, Eliza, was three, she offered me a moment of awe before bedtime: "Mommy, you know what? If you believe in yourself and close your eyes, you see a light!" To this day, I marvel at how she came up with that piece of wisdom.

As you continue to interact with others, whether they are living with dementia or other challenges life has embedded in their path, please cherish your belief in yourself. Trust the shining light of your ability to care and to love. I wish you joy, peace and strength on the journey.

Thank you for reading *Looking Past Dementia*.
If you've enjoyed this book, please leave a review on your favorite review site. In doing so, you can help equip other readers to experience more joy, connection, love, laughter and engagement with those living with dementia.

Appendix A. Strategies for Managing (or Reducing the Risk of) Dementia

Many people ask whether there are ways to reduce the risk of dementia. While no strategy can guarantee prevention, growing research indicates that certain lifestyle habits support brain health and overall well-being. These activities enrich our lives regardless of age or diagnosis by keeping us connected, engaged, active and emotionally supported.

1. **Exercise.** Exercise is at the top of the list for maintaining brain health. It is believed to be the single best thing we can do for our brains. If you're unsure about suitable activities for you or your loved one, consult your doctor for guidance.
2. **Focus on eating habits.** A plant-based, organic diet is not just a suggestion; it's a fundamental key to wellness. Ensure you drink enough water, limit sugar intake, and include Omega 3-rich fats in your diet (found in nuts, seeds and fatty fish, like salmon, rainbow trout, and lake whitefish).

3. **Reduce your stress.** Devote plenty of time to things that help you relax and give you joy. One possibility would be listening to your favorite music for thirty minutes daily.
4. **Maintain a sense of purpose, meaning and engagement.** It's important to stay involved in tasks you love and to show your care for others. We all need opportunities to make a difference.
5. **Get 7–8 hours of sleep each night. This** is vital for protecting brain health and managing dementia. Avoid consuming caffeine in the afternoon or evening to improve your sleep quality.
6. **Learn new things.** Complexity grows the brain. New interests can be developed, and creative pursuits can be adapted to suit our abilities as we age.
7. **Stay engaged.** As social creatures, we need to interact and be in community with others for our mental health as well as our brain health.
8. **Humor is healing.** We should do whatever we can to bring more humor into our lives. A moment of laughter can reduce stress, lift spirits, and help people feel more connected to one another.[37]

37 The author gratefully acknowledges the Dementia Action Alliance, including Laurie Scherrer, Janice Bays, and Casey Venturini, for their inspiration and guidance related to the ideas presented in this appendix.

Appendix B. Making the Move to Memory Care

Moving a loved one into memory care is often an emotional and complicated process for everyone involved. Families may struggle with questions about safety, timing, independence and quality of life, while the individual living with dementia may feel confused, frightened, resistant or even relieved. So, when is it the right time to move? And how do we do this?

There is no one-size-fits-all answer to these questions. It depends on the individual and the stage of their dementia progression. Do they understand they have cognitive issues, or are they unaware they are living with dementia? Is their current environment safe and supportive enough for their needs? How quickly does the person seem to be advancing?

Signs that it may be time include:

- episodes of wandering away from safety or getting lost
- poor hygiene
- medication mix-ups
- difficulty socializing or avoiding others
- changed eating habits or weight loss
- decline in overall well-being
- increased caregiver strain or burnout

If an individual clearly needs more structure, engagement and direction, an adult day program is a wonderful transitional step toward memory care and allows them to live longer in their home while giving you a much-needed break.

There are various approaches you can use when discussing the need to transition someone to memory care. But no matter what, don't just take them, drop them off, and leave. (Yes, sadly, that happens.) And it's also better not to inform the person weeks in advance. Instead, consider using one of these options:

- Some people take the person out to lunch at the residence once or twice, and then, having already moved their belongings, show them their new room: "Surprise!" This can be an effective option, though it may not be particularly pleasant for some. Still, people can and do adjust.
- Engage the person's physician to gain their support. If the individual being moved trusts them, perhaps the doctor could deliver the initial message.
- If you are comfortable with therapeutic fibbing, carefully chosen white lies can sometimes ease the transition. Dementia care expert and educator Rachael Wonderlin offers three things to say that can be helpful:
  - **Blame the doctor:** "The doctor wants you to go here."
  - **Name a vague length of time:** "for a little while" or "for a few months."
  - **Give a plausible reason** (unrelated to dementia): "so they can better monitor your new medication," "while your leg heals," or "for your arthritis."[38]

38 Rachael Wonderlin, "The 3 best things to say when transitioning someone to a dementia care community," YouTube video, January 5, 2022, emeraldlakebooks.com/wonderlin.

- Alternatively, saying "Your house has mold in it and it's going to take some time to get that fixed" worked very well for one family I knew to convince Mom to move into assisted living.
- Another alternative… Tell the truth (what a concept!), especially if the person is aware of their cognitive decline and is able to reason. "The doctor thinks we should try this place out, and that it might be good for you to get a little extra care right now."
- Is there anything your relative used to say to you that could be useful in this situation? "You always told me, Mom, that sometimes life is hard, but we get through, and we can adjust."

In discussions regarding an upcoming move, avoid arguing or attempting to persuade. Tread lightly, speak softly and clearly, and be patient.

Regardless of how the transition unfolds, people generally settle in and adapt. This process typically takes anywhere from three weeks to three months. Here are a few things you can do to make the transition easier for your loved one:

- Visit the selected community with the individual who will be relocating multiple times before moving day. Have lunch there or participate in an activity.
- Make their new environment as much like their current home as possible. Work with a moving company that understands memory care needs.
- Validate the person's feelings: "Dad, if I were you, I would feel the same way." "I know, this is hard." "I'm so sorry, Mom. I wish things were different."

Once you have moved your relative, consider participating in the life of the community, especially during those first few days and weeks. Attend events and activities with your loved one or share a meal together. If you have time to volunteer by playing the piano or showcasing another special talent, or if you can help lead an activity that highlights something amazing your family member accomplished in their life, speak with the activities director or memory care coordinator about making that happen.

Acknowledgments

Bringing a book into being is a collaborative process, not unlike launching a theater production. Lots of individuals are involved, many behind the scenes, each playing a separate yet vitally important part.

The book, star of a one-person show, is currently pacing in the wings as I write this, waiting for necessary elements to be spliced together for opening night. As the author, I'm the overly protective stage mother, juggling last-minute details and pushing assigned tasks toward completion, while trying to calm my nerves concerning how my child will fare when the curtain finally rises. Fortunately, books don't forget their lines.

My first large parcel of gratitude goes to Jill Nokleby Kaiser, who hired me in 2003 with the imagination necessary to consider my theater experience a suitable backdrop for working in memory care. Without her confidence, I would not have enjoyed twelve years of knowing the individuals who, decades later, would become actors on the stage of my manuscript. Other professionals I must thank for their belief in me include Candace Gislason, Julie Thurn, Jon Lundberg, Ann Schrempp, Mike Ziomko, Brendan Bannigan, Barbara Mekenye, Brenda Johnson, and Terri Bates, all from Ebenezer Management Services. Additional thanks belong to Patti Knutson, Scott Saffert, Susan Snyder, and Lori McGuire from my time working at The Glenn Hopkins, and to Awa Sey Yaffa for approving the story in which she played an integral part.

Enormous kudos to my brilliant publisher, Tara R. Alemany from Emerald Lake Books, the director of this project, along with her cast of editors, designers, proofreaders and other assistants who have contributed to making my book ever so much better. Tara, exceedingly skilled, is a tireless worker and an expert communicator. She has been helpful and patient with my questions, doubts, foibles and occasional angst.

I am indebted to my manuscript's first audience of readers: poet Zoë Bird and authors Pamela Joern and Megan Carnarius—all skilled creative writers. Each of them gave me incisive, encouraging notes to consider. Author and playwright Jenna Zark combed an early edition of my manuscript with her copy editor's eye. She quickly won my trust and became a friend. I doubt my manuscript would have received interest from a publisher without her proficiency.

Friends have been essential along the way to opening night. I cannot fathom how I would have managed without the balm of relationship and enthusiasm supplied by my decades-long Women's Group and others with whom I speak, dine, write, drink coffee and tea, see plays or movies, and celebrate with. I am grateful also to my loyal tribe of interested high school friends (you know who you are!), scattered across the country, who contributed mightily to my love of drama, humor, words, people, laughter and life itself.

Phillipa Anastos, George Anastos, and Walton Stanley, you were right there for me at critical times when I needed technical help.

A special shout-out to my writing group, the Soapstone Writers Collective—Sarah Koper, Robert McClain, Rachel Clark, and Betty Goihl—for inspiration and reassurance.

Big thanks also to my family—my daughter Eliza Swanson, sister Marilyn Moses, brother Bob Moses, nephews Stephen and David Warch, and niece Karin Warch. I am grateful to you all for your interested, encouragement, skills, generosity, kindness and unwavering support.

This book would not exist without my mother, Margaret Moses, and others living with dementia who taught me so much. I am also deeply grateful to family and friends long gone, each of whom made an indelible, dramatic impression on me. My grandmothers, Lois M. Gemeny and LaVere Coleman, were both attuned to the arts and wrote poetry. My grandad, James P. Coleman, and my uncle, Bob Coleman, were delightfully clever and prolific in their correspondence. I still miss my conscientious father, C. Everett Moses (another prolific letter writer); my loving and gifted sisters, Margot Warch and Lois Moses; my brilliant brother-in-law, Rik Warch (who, when I was about four years old, dutifully watched my made-up plays while waiting for Margot to finish getting ready for their dates); my mild-mannered, yet groundbreaking drama teacher, Jack Boyle; my unusually talented friends, Michael Macmacha and Chris Armstrong; and of course, the irreplaceable, inimitable Phil Kilbourne—my husband, laugh-inducer and love of my life.

Grateful applause to all mentioned here!

About the Author

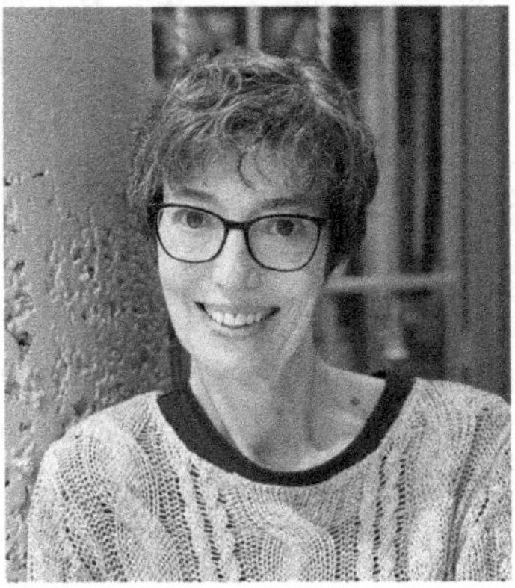

Marysue Moses is a dementia educator, consultant and former memory care coordinator who has spent years helping caregivers and professionals create more meaningful, engaging experiences for people living with dementia.

Long before she entered the field of dementia care, Marysue was a theater artist. A self-described "theater kid" who studied in London, worked with the Illusion Theater in Minneapolis, and co-founded Theatre at Work, she developed a deep appreciation for storytelling, presence and human connection—skills that would later shape her approach to dementia care in unexpected ways.

Her path into that work began with her mother's dementia diagnosis. As she tried to better understand what her mother was experiencing, she was struck by the lack of meaningful engagement in many memory care settings. Drawing on her theatrical background, she created Tales from a Trunk, an interactive storytelling program that uses props and sensory experiences to spark connection and invite participation. What began as a way to serve her own family quickly grew into a broader calling.

Marysue went on to work in an assisted living community as an activities coordinator and then as a memory care coordinator while earning her master's degree in gerontology. She later served as the dementia program coordinator for Ebenezer Management Services, where she helped develop training and best practices across multiple sites. Today, she continues her work as a dementia educator, sharing practical, creative approaches with caregivers, families and professionals across the country.

Family has remained at the heart of Marysue's work and perspective. She was married to actor Phil Kilbourne, whose curiosity and encouragement supported her journey, and she is the proud mother of a creative and enterprising daughter. The people she has loved—both at home and in her care communities—continue to shape the way she teaches, writes and connects with others.

If you're interested in having Marysue speak to your group or organization, you can contact her at emeraldlakebooks.com/moses.

www.ingramcontent.com/pod-product-compliance
Lightning Source LLC
LaVergne TN
LVHW010720061126
851857LV00014B/1269
* 9 7 8 1 9 4 5 8 4 7 9 6 7 *